Fun and Laughter in Recovery,

Otherwise, Why Recover?

Ronald Lee Cobb

Fun and Laughter in Recovery / Ronald Lee Cobb

Fun and Laughter in Recovery, Otherwise, Why Recover?

Meeting God Day by Day, by Lynne Chandler (2014, Forward Movement) reprinted by permission.

PRINTED IN THE U.S.A.

DEDICATION

This book on fun and laughter and recovery is dedicated to Betty Kooser Letterman. Betty personifies the tough stance this book takes on daily deciding to intentionally live out fun and laughter even amid the struggles and vicissitudes of life. Betty has experienced many of the difficult things mentioned in the dozens of stories in this book: serious illnesses, the loss of her husband, extremely painful issues with those for whom she really cares, and yet, year after year, day after day, she cognitively makes the decision to be positive, caring, and even full of fun and play during some of her darkest hours. Everyone who knows Betty well loves Betty. Few people inspire me like she does. Betty Kooser Letterman, thank you for being in my life.

TABLE of CONTENTS

PREFACE

The fun and laughter described in this book can be surprisingly powerful. Such a daily, healthy lifestyle can bring monumental healing to every human heart. It can help a person recover more quickly from physical illness, emotional pain, psychological imbalance, trauma, substance abuse, and spiritual injuries.

The intent of this book is to help every reader make the decision to begin a journey to live out the therapeutic wisdom of *deciding* to enjoy life. Writing in the February 22nd 2016 edition of *Time Magazine,* Mary Oaklander quotes Dr. Sarah Pressman, of the University of California, who has been researching happiness for about a decade. "Positive emotion is good for you.'" Oaklander goes on to say, "Her experiments have found that people who smiled while receiving a needle injection rated the ordeal as 40% less painful than those who did not smile…their heart rates did not increase as much in response to the stress of the injection, either."

She quotes Dr. Pressman as then saying, "Now when I go to the doctor's office I smile when I get a shot."

I hope the positive stories in this book also ease your pain as you read these words. May they encourage you to gain the ability to laugh even during pain, and to have peaceful fun and joy and assurance, even in the midst of the deepest sorrow.

It is clear in their teachings that Isaiah, Buddha, Marcus Aurelius, Jesus of Nazareth, Rumi, Mahatma Gandhi, Martin Luther King, and the great teachers throughout the ages, had a deep sense of fun and fulfillment throughout their lives. They were doing what they were created to do, at times showing subtle, whimsical laughter, or even straightforward humor during their most epic struggles.

Sincere thanks to Esther Luttrell for encouraging me as I wrote this book and for helping me with the details of publishing, and to Duane Hermann for his wise and helpful comments as he proofread the book.

1

Cancer, a Colostomy Bag
and Still Having Fun
and Laughter in Recovery

Betty Letterman is a vivacious, fun-to-be-with friend. My wife and I love to be around her. She is physically active, cheerful, and has a very positive outlook on life. She is a dedicated church member and a hard worker. One day she told me part of her life story. I was amazed at her resilience as she spilled out the details of her personal history.

As a young adult she had drunk a lot of alcohol. She had been addicted to cigarettes. She had also become addicted to food. It was a trifecta of three dangerous addictions. She began having severe pain and went for medical help. Her doctor found a two inch cancer in her colon.

She quit drinking and quit smoking cigarettes, and lost 100 lbs. Most of her colon was surgically removed. She was given a colostomy bag.

"I knew that for my own mental health I needed to give that bag a name so I called him Willard," she said.

I told Betty that I had known others who had given parts of their body a name, but Betty was the only person I had ever known to name her colostomy bag. We both laughed.

What an incredible stance. What a positive mental health maneuver, to enjoy life and laugh in the face of her own recovery from cancer. For the past 22 years she has sent birthday cards and Christmas cards to her family and friends, ending with the words, "Love, Betty and Willard."

Betty has a deep faith in God. She began realizing that, for years after her surgery, she was an untreated dry alcoholic and a dry nicotine addict and an untreated food addict.

I admire Betty's deep fun and laughter in her recovery, in spite of her struggles, pain, and trials.

When I grow up I want to be like Betty.

2

A New Concept:
Being Able to Remember
Everything at the Dance

One of my friends had abused drugs and alcohol throughout his teen years and came to treatment in his mid-twenties. A Narcotics Anonymous dance was coming up and I encouraged him to attend. "I can't go," he said. He was a normal, active, intelligent young adult and his reply startled me. "I can't go because I have never danced clean and sober. I have always gone to dances high from drugs or buzzed from alcohol. I can't dance unless I am high on something."

I told him that dancing was like learning how to ride a bicycle; once you learn how to do it you over-learned it and could easily do it again, even if you had not ridden a bicycle for years. I told him he would be fine. He went to the dance, but he was really worried.

It was so much fun to see him return.

"I did it! I did it! I danced clean and sober. It was fun, I had a blast, and I can remember everything." He was so happy he was literally jumping up and down and his smile was a foot wide.

He was beginning to discover fun and laughter in recovery even though he was still in his post-acute withdrawal phase of healing from his years of substance abuse.

3

To Have Fun and Laughter is a Daily Decision

The first time I heard that "love is a decision" it did not make sense to me. Love was an emotion. How could it be a decision?

Over the years I came to realize that we can indeed decide to love ourselves and to love other people. It is a decision. It is easy to decide to love those we like and are attracted to. It is more difficult to love those we don't like, but we can even make a decision to do that.

Jesus commanded us to love our enemies. He did not tell us to like them. He told us to love them. One secret is that in learning to love everyone, including our enemies, we learn to love ourselves, for often we are our own worst enemy.

In a similar manner we need to make the decision every day to have fun and laughter in recovery. Sometimes fun and laughter are spontaneous, but persons with substance abuse, physical health issues, and mental health disorder histories need to make a conscious, cognitive decision every day to have fun, to have laughter, and to love. The three are all related.

I have friend who, every time he goes to work, has fun and laughs a lot. He told me that he had cognitively decided to make this positive way of living part of his recovery. "I have to work and make a living," he said. "So I decided I am going to have fun at work every day."

Needless to say people enjoy hanging out with my friend. He is an inspiration. I try to follow his example every single day.

4

Medical Wisdom
about Laughter and Humor
in the Mayo Clinic Newsletter

July 2015 issue of the Mayo Clinic newsletter (*www.HealthLetter.MayoClinic.com*) pointed out that "Laughter is a physical action that... involves flexing of facial muscles, powerful contractions of the diaphragm, repetitive voice sounds, and other body movements such as swaying or clapping—and sometimes even tears."

In other words, hearty laughter is a mini-workout of sorts. Your heart rate, breathing rate, oxygen consumption and calorie burn all rise when laughing—muscles throughout the body are worked.

The Mayo article pointed out that finding humor in stressful situations had "stress-relieving benefits." Not only does humor have stress-relieving benefits, but "it can serve as a bonding mechanism in groups... increases one's likeability... and be an important component of avoiding loneliness and social isolation."

Loneliness and social isolation are the dangerous realities of long-term mental health disorders and long-term alcohol or drug abuse.

The article points out that taking life too seriously can become a handicap and that it is important to "spend time with friends who make you laugh. Maybe you contribute with a joke or story of your own, or maybe you just contribute by laughing."

It other words make a cognitive decision to laugh and enjoy life.

5

Healing Benefits of Fun and Laughter

Cancer Centers of America have published the following benefits of laughter. The list they have developed shows the physical benefits, mental benefits, and psychological benefits of laughter. In other words, fun and laughter in recovery will help you become a whole person again. Cancer Centers of America calls it "Laughter Therapy."

- Boost the immune system and circulatory system
- Enhance oxygen intake
- Stimulate the heart and lungs
- Relax muscles throughout the body
- Trigger the release of endorphins (the body's natural painkillers)
- Ease digestion/soothes stomach aches
- Relieve pain
- Balance blood pressure
- Improve mental functions (i.e., alertness, memory, creativity)

Laughter therapy may also help to:

- Improve overall attitude
- Reduce stress/tension
- Promote relaxation
- Improve sleep
- Enhance quality of life
- Strengthen social bonds and relationships
- Produce a general sense of well-being

6

The Human Brain
and
Fun and Laughter in Recovery

After the darkness and depression of substance abuse or trauma, or health related problems, having fun and laughter in recovery are essential for long-term overall health.

It sometimes takes the brain at least a year of clean time to develop positive beta-endorphin levels, more normal serotonin levels, and a myriad of other complex systems. This means, that during the first year of recovery from any illness, waves of positive emotions and of negative emotions return in full force, and there are no pain meds, anxiety meds, pot, meth, cocaine, alcohol or other addictive behaviors to hide from them.

Getting through this difficult period without relapsing on substances or relapsing into negative mental health issues is foundational.

Fun and laughter are essential in early recovery, in the middle stages of recovery, and then they need to continue to last throughout a recovering person's entire lifetime.

7

Fun and Laughter
Reduces Cortisol and Stress

Christopher Bergland, writing in *The Athlete's Way* on January 22, 2013, found that "cortisol is released in response to fear or stress by the adrenal glands as part of the flight-or-flight syndrome. Once the alarm to release cortisol has sounded, your body becomes mobilized and ready for action, but there has to be a physical release of fight or flight, otherwise, cortisol levels build up in the blood. This cortisol then wreaks havoc on your mind and body."

Physical exercise, or completing a difficult task, will cause cortisol levels to return to normal. Again, quoting Bergland, "Distress, or free floating anxiety, doesn't provide an outlet for the cortisol." Bergland believes that cortisol is "public enemy number one" because "scientists have known for years that elevated cortisol levels interfere with learning, memory, lower immune function, lower bone density, increased weight gain, blood pressure, cholesterol, heart disease, depression, mental illness, lower life expectancy, and the list goes on and on."

What does a recovering person need to do to deal with stress?

They must first learn to talk about their stress with people who love them and who understand. They need to take steps to deal with their stress physically by moderate physical exercise.

Helping other people in recovery is one of the hidden healing suggestions in the 12 Steps.

Get the focus off of yourself, refuse to think about your own stress, and reach out with love and care for others. This will automatically lead you to more fully love and care for yourself, and allow you to experience more healing laughter and fun.

8

Fun and Laughter
and the Need for Being
with Positive, Recovering People

Isolation is co-morbid with physical pain issues, depression, addiction and other related mental health disorders. There can be social isolation behaviors, physical isolation, emotional isolation, spiritual isolation, psychological isolation, and mental isolation.

Fun and laughter are just the opposite of isolation.

We need other people in our recovery. It is fine to have fun and laughter in recovery by ourselves, but fun and laughter are more than doubled when we have fun and laughter with others.

Fun and laughter do not always just suddenly appear. We often have to make them happen. We cannot sit around waiting for someone to invite us to do something fun.

Early in my recovery I began to realize that I was the one who needed to get off of dead center after a lifetime of isolation and depression.

9

Making a List of Friends Who Like Fun and Laughter

I developed lists of persons who liked to canoe, who liked to camp out, who liked to hike, who liked to go to worship services, who liked to go to support group meetings, who liked to play tennis, who liked to study interesting books and concepts, or who liked to play golf.

I did not wait for others to call me. When I was lonely I called other recovering persons. I systematically called one phone number after another until I found someone who was able to schedule a fun time with me.

The word "recreation" means we can "recreate" our lives. Recreation, fun, and laughter mold us into the kind of human being that other people want to be with.

Fun and laughter in recovery at its highest level is essentially self-originated, self-actualized, and self-motivated behavior. This is the best kind of fun and laughter, self-actualized fun and laughter in doing things that are not addictive.

It is living out the proverb, "The best things in life are free."

10

The Importance of Laughing Out Loud

Give yourself permission to laugh out loud. I would suggest that you do not settle for quiet snickers or muffled smiles. Allow yourself to laugh wholeheartedly with gusto.

Many scientific studies have shown that laughter is healing. Norman Cousins wrote a book, *Anatomy of an Illness.* He had been diagnosed with a fast-growing terminal cancer and was told that he did not have very long to live, but Norman had a theory he wanted to prove. He theorized that laughing and having fun were healing.

Norman's story took place many years ago before cell phones, or even 8mm films, were available for private use. He was a very successful writer, with a lot of money, so he made a small theater in his home and purchased 16mm films of cartoons that made him laugh. Every day he watched mindless, funny cartoons like *Tom and Jerry*, and gave himself permission to laugh out loud.

Norman lived ten years longer than his cancer doctor predicted, and he had the added bonus of having fun and laughter during almost every single day of every one of those ten years.

11

Systematic Physical Exercise and Fun and Laughter: the "Fountain of Youth"

Physical exercise is a very important area of recovery. We just discussed how physical activities like dancing, canoeing, tennis, hiking, etc. help a person have fun and laughter in recovery.

Making systematic physical endeavors enjoyable can help a person have fun and laughter in recovery in a way that causes holistic and comprehensive regeneration as nothing else can.

When I was writing my doctoral dissertation on senior adults, I studied the results of dozens of medical studies on older Americans. Over and over again these studies led me to find the proverbial "Fountain of Youth."

The fountain of youth is regular, consistent aerobic exercise.

It is important to find several exercises you enjoy (to maintain the fun and laughter). *Several* different sets of exercise regimens are important, because you need to cross-train every part of your body.

Exercise gives one a natural high.

12

Natural Highs, Weight Lifting,
Even Legal Things
Can Lead to Recovery

Attending a helpful worship service, a positive Alcoholics Anonymous meeting, seeing a good movie, or any fun event of kind, can give you a natural high just like physical exercise gives you a high. It is long lasting high that is beneficial to your long-term recovery.

As a youth I could not understand why I liked weight-lifting so much. Later, in my doctoral studies, I learned that weight-lifting gives a person several times more of an endorphin "rush" than any other exercise. It is legal. It is healthy. It is fun.

People often drink alcohol or use drugs to self-medicate mental health issues, trauma issues, or pain issues, in an artificial endeavor to have fun and laughter. Weight-lifting is a natural way of getting "high" and having fun and laughter.

As an adolescent I struggled with depression and I found that when I lifted weights, I felt much less depression and, therefore, much less of a need for "living on the edge" or artificial highs.

My doctoral studies uncovered studies of senior adults who were regular weight-lifters. These studies even more deeply ingrained my insights in this area. One medical study took 100 healthy senior adults and measured their bone density. Then the study measured the bone density of 100 other healthy senior adults. The first 100 seniors agreed to a moderate weight-lifting regimen while the second group of 100 just lived a normal life. At the end of the year the study tested the bone density of the first 100 moderate weight-lifters and found that they had gained 2.7% more bone density. When the sedentary seniors were tested they had lost 3.3% bone density.

Something else the study did not mention was that the weight-lifting group had a better sense of balance, better appetite, an increased overall health, and better brain function.

Numerous studies have shown that drugs and alcohol cause one to have a lack of proper nutrition. In senior adults, lack of oxygen to the brain can be the result of not exercising. Numerous studies of senior adults have found that seniors who regularly exercise do not have significant brain shrinkage. Their thought processes were much less compromised.

I am also sure that the weight-lifting group also had more fun and laughter, with their increased mental capabilities and their enhanced physical well-being.

Choose other exercises that you like, whether it is yoga, tai-chi, weightlifting, long walks, dancing, moderate gymnastics, etc. One thing to be careful about is that persons with mental health issues, and with substance abuse issues, can become addicted to over-exercise. Over-exercise does not give the body time to regenerate after vigorous workouts, and can produce the opposite effect, diminishing fun and laughter in recovery and increasing pain.

Addicts tend to think if something is good then a whole lot of it must be very good, but this does not hold true for exercise or for any other excesses. Moderation is the key to a higher quality of fun and laughter in recovery.

13

Non-Physical Fun and Laughter in Recovery

Fun does not always have to be physically related. There is incredible joy in slowing down and watching the sun magnificently rise in the east or peacefully set in a beautiful sunset. Peaceful fun can be just as healing as boisterous fun. Reading a true love story works. Watching a non-violent, peaceful movie can work. One fun thing I do every morning and every evening is to feed the deer, wild turkeys, squirrels, song birds, and barn cat.

As I was typing this particular chapter, four buzzards landed on the silo by our barn. They spread their wings in the sunlight, drying them from the wet dew of the spring morning. Soon they flew off to begin cleaning the earth. As I was later writing down these words, I saw a doe came out of the woods to eat the corn offering I had left for her. A squirrel was sitting next to her on the corn that was spread out on the low concrete table. They were sharing the same meal. They left and were followed by a young raccoon eating until he was full.

Deep fun like this and soul joy in peaceful settings like this are things that every human being need, to be inwardly nourished.

Persons recovering from physical illnesses, with substance abuse issues, or with mental health disorders, especially need peace to stay alive and to flourish because, frequently, negative issues can grow together in a co-morbid manner, festering from feeding off of each other.

Fun and laughter are not simply survival skills, but skills that can be used to become fully self-actualized, fulfilled persons.

Fun and laughter are a foundational essence of recovery and one of its greatest benefits.

14

Quiet Fun and Laughter
Simply Reading in a Corner of the Room

Elizabeth was so much different from her brother. Her metabolism did not force her to run and skip and jump like her brother. From the minute she learned to read, she could sit in the corner of a room and quietly read, and she loved to read.

Some of her prose poems in grade school were incredibly profound. People who like to read generally tend to be good writers because of their familiarity with several authors and their knowledge of different styles of writing.

There was one particular family we would visit before my daughter, Elizabeth, was born that had so much chaos and activity going on in their home the only way I could stay sane was to go off in a corner of their living room and read interesting magazine articles. They never said anything about it directly to me. To keep myself internally grounded and peaceful, I continued to read rather than get involved in that family's rather intense interactions and negative humor that put other people down.

Years later, when Elizabeth was part of this family as a teenager; she did not know any of my past reading-to-survive-in-chaos behaviors, and she did the same thing.

One of the family members confronted her. "All you ever do is read. You don't enter into our (chaotic) discussions. You are just like your father," the person said.

Their criticism surprised Elizabeth. They liked David, her brother. He was loud and boisterous and gregarious and joined right in with their kidding, chaotic interactions. Elizabeth had fun just sitting quietly and reading a good book. Her laughter was internalized.

Every one experiences fun and laughter in different ways. It is important to give everyone their own space in finding their own comfort zone of fun and laughter.

15

"What if?" Thinking is the Opposite of Fun and Laughter

A frequent robber of fun and laughter is "what if?" thinking. "What if?" is a poison to fun and laughter, and needs to be avoided like the bubonic plague.

Just the words "what if?" cause fear and anxiety to arise. So many soldiers were terrified of leaving the concrete and steel walls of Eagle Base to enjoy the country. "What if we get ambushed? What if we hit a land mine?"

When we would create war contingency plans in the Army, we would war-game from the lowest problem to the highest problem, but we did not live in any of those "what if?" plans. We were simply ready for anything that developed.

It is okay to plan for the future. It is not okay to emotionally live in the "what if?" future.

Often people in early recovery get trapped in this negative thinking. They begin to worry about everything in the past and everything that may happen in the future. Fear and anxiety like this are almost always associated with anxiety and depression, and depression is the farthest thing from fun and laughter. Depression can lead right back to unbalanced mental health, inappropriate anger, and can often lead to substance abuse.

Peace and serenity are the fruits of recovery. This is why the concept of a loving higher power is so important in every one of the 12 Steps and why it is important to have fun and laughter in individual recovery.

16

The Concept of a Higher Power, Acceptance, and Fun and Laughter

When you know that you belong in the world, and that you are a child of God, the world becomes a safer place.

I had been practicing fun and laughter in recovery for several years when I was called to active duty in a hostile fire zone. Some of the areas around Eagle Base were not the safest places to be, yet years of working the 12 Steps—which are inherently spiritual by their nature—gave me a very helpful antidote to fear and to "what if?" thinking. I refused to do negative, harmful "what if?" speculation on the convoys and missions I was on.

"Acceptance is the answer to all my problems" is one of the most profound sentences in the AA "Big Book." Acceptance is the answer to "what if?" thinking.

A personal relationship with a higher power helps a person find genuine inner peace and therefore liberates a person to actually experience fun and laughter in recovery. There was a saying we had at Menninger Psychiatric Hospital in our addictions work: "Without spiritual recovery there is no recovery." Related to this is a profound statement Karl Menninger made many years ago: "Long before there was psychology or psychiatry there was a faith in God. A faith in God has helped keep people sane for thousands of years."

Fun and laughter, and a faith in a loving Higher Power, not only helps keep us sane, it also helps us to not take ourselves so seriously.

17

The Best Fun and Laughter
We Can Experience is to
Make Fun of Ourselves

As a young professional, I spent several days in Upstate New York and in New York City with Dr. Norman Vincent Peale and his wife Ruth. I noticed that he had a great deal of fun and laughter both during his small talk with others individually and, also, in his more formal public presentations. He would make jokes about his own errors and weaknesses, and everyone one of us loved him because we had similar *faux pas* in our own lives. He never once made fun of other people, just himself.

At one of our meetings a colleague of Dr. Peale stood up and told a joke. The joke centered on how he felt like he was stuck in a hen house and his wife was pecking him to death. It was a funny joke, but it was also a passive-aggressive put-down of his wife. When Dr. Peale stood up to follow him, he kindly, gently, responded, "Now John, I know your wife. She is a fine lady and her fried chicken is the best I have ever eaten."

President Harry Truman never took himself too seriously and told jokes about himself on a regular basis. Truman would tell how his wife had to work with him to not use words that would be offensive to others. He was taking some high society women on a tour of the garden by the White House. They asked him what they used to fertilize the plants. Truman said he used the word "manure." Afterwards one of the high society matrons told the President's wife Beth, "Your husband said they used 'manure' to fertilize the plants." Beth had a good supply of fun and laughter herself and she laughingly replied, "Oh thank goodness he did not use that other word."

Having fun and laughter in recovery helps us learn how to joke about our own shortcomings and weaknesses, and not to take ourselves so seriously. When a person takes themselves seriously all the time, they tend to act like a "dry drunk", or a "dry addict", or a person with an untreated mental health disorder such as narcissism. They think that every time they utter an opinion they are speaking *ex cathedra* like a Pope.

So many of my untreated friends have spoken bombastically like this; I have seen it so often that I never want to go there. I'd rather make fun of myself and then to allow myself to laugh wholeheartedly at myself, and never make fun of other people.

18

Creative Spirituality from Cairo, Egypt, a Humorous yet Insightful Story

*I*t had become a tradition to release a dove in our church garden in Cairo, Egypt, at the end of Pentecost Day (When churches worldwide celebrate the day the Spirit of God descended on the early Christians). Our church used a white homing pigeon that was able to fly straight home to avoid the city hawks on its route.

One year, on the eve of Pentecost Day, my daughter rushed into our room in a panic. "Where's the Pentecost bird?" she wanted to know.

We found our big, gentle dog, Pepsi, cowering in the corner. Feathers were strewn everywhere. The bird's box was tipped over; it was gone. Could our pampered pet have annihilated an ancient Christian symbol?

We finally found the little winged creature, hiding in a corner, not long for this world. I cried. How could I possibly face our congregation with such news? Thankfully, Cairo is a place where a replacement can be found even in the night culture of Egypt, so I sent my husband out into the darkness to search. (He did find a replacement and being gone some time.)

I knew he would have to climb dark, rickety stairs to reach a rooftop loft. Cairo is full of hundreds of such pigeon lofts. Earlier, I had watched a man exercising his rooftop pigeons, whistling signals and waving a white flag. His pigeons flew freely and powerfully. When he eventually called them home, he must have watched them with such joy and pride as they *returned to their loft. He was having such fun and fulfillment in raising them. A bird like his would rescue Pentecost.*

The Spirit's descent into our lives arrives on the wings of hope and joy, and offers a presence as intimate as our very own breath—divine and mysterious, full of life-giving strength to sustain us.

(Adapted from Lynne Chandler's words, page 150, *Meeting God Day by Day*, 2014, Forward Movement)

19

Loving Your Work
and Working for Love

O n many occasions I have worked with people who have stated, "I hate my work. I hate getting up in the morning." We would then discuss how this hatred of their work was precisely what had brought them to my clinic office for individual therapy. We discussed what were some of things they enjoyed doing at work and how doing something they love would help them work from a center of fun and laughter and love.

If they could find this new stance would then a dramatic paradigm shift took place and their universe changed. They would want to get up in the morning. They would love the people they were helping. They would love the details of their work. They would love life. Most importantly, they would begin to love themselves, because now they were operating from love.

I have a friend who is a retired psychiatrist. He loves to do intricate, beautiful wood carvings. They are awesome creations, but best of all, he is full of love and he is full of life. He is experiencing fun and laughter in recovery and is being healed from his many past traumas of having to deal with agonizing volumes of human suffering that people in his field must, of necessity, daily face.

I used to enjoy seeing my pre-school son run for the sheer enjoyment of being alive. My friend is now carving wood for sheer enjoyment.

Fun and laughter helps us become fully alive.

20

Fun and Laughter at Work?
Is it Possible?

People who hate to go to work, or dislike what they are doing, often become my patients because their anger, hatreds, and resentments about their job are driving them to alcohol or drugs or exacerbating their pre-existing mental health disorders. My advice? Find a job you like and make a decision to have fun and laughter at work every day.

I have heard many reasons for hating jobs:

"I went to school to learn how to do this. I don't like it anymore."

"I can't quit this job. I'm making a lot of money."

"I never did want to be in this family business."

My advice has always been to quit their job after they have find a job they would really like. When you are doing work you love doing, you really are not working; it is like getting paid to do a hobby that you love, like carving birds. You are on vacation.

I have followed my own advice several times and quit working at jobs that were destroying me emotionally, going against my ethics, or in other ways harming me.

"But I will lose a lot of money," people consistently me. My response has been that, if they continue to force themselves to work at a job they intensely dislike, they will again become a patient in a clinic or hospital, costing more money and pain.

Money is secondary. Are you doing what you like? Do you have a job you love? A person who has a job they love is very rich. Living a life of love and fun and laughter need to be in everything recovering people do, including their daily job.

Starting out in the work-a-day world, it is often necessary to have an entry level job that is not so pleasant, but "this too shall pass." If you are working toward the goal of doing something you love body, soul, mind, and spirit, you will become more and happy as you make steady progress in finding that joy.

21

The Decision of Martin Luther
to Move His Life
from Despair to Rejoicing

Billy Graham, in his book, *Hope for Each Day* (pg 170), tells a little known story of how Martin Luther, beset with much opposition and many problems after the Reformation began, went through a very difficult period in his life. Dr. Graham writes, "One day his wife came to the breakfast table all dressed in black, as if she were going to a funeral service. When Martin asked her who had died, she replied, 'Martin, the way you've been behaving lately, I thought God had died, so I came prepared to attend His funeral'."

Martin Luther saw his wife's object lesson and heeded her gentle advice. This great "reformer resolved to never again to allow worldly care, resentment, depression, discouragement, or frustration defeat him. By God's grace, he vowed he would submit his life to the God and reflect his grace in a spirit of rejoicing."

Martin Luther did a paradigm shift by making the decision to rejoice and to have fun and laughter in his life regardless of his circumstances. He made the decision to be positive and upbeat and to have a joyful attitude. Thus he began to inspire his children, his wife, his church and his offspring still live in eastern Germany.

What would have happened if he had allowed his depression to conquer him?

You and I can make the same decision to have fun and laughter in our lives, regardless of any other negative circumstances.

22

People Who Have Fun and Laughter are No Longer Victims!

Have you ever noticed that some people who take themselves very seriously rarely laugh or appear to be having fun? Some of them seem to believe that every word they speak has the gravity of absolute truth and law, as mentioned earlier. These poor folks need to lighten up. One needs to constantly realize they are a fallible, imperfect human being and to learn to heartily laugh and have more fun.

People in long-term recovery from physical illnesses, substance abuse, and mental health disorders, can also learn how to enjoy life by being less obsessive-compulsive. One big relapse warning sign is perfectionism. Often perfectionists try to control every person and everything around them. This impossible dream only leads them to become more of a victim. It leads to feelings of anger, defeat, and to the very edge of relapse. There is no way you can control every other person and everything. Thus they can lapse into victimhood.

Victims are powerless. Many people like the victim role because they don't have to do anything. It is everyone else's fault. They often never find full recovery because victims live in a "poor me" world.

People in recovery learn to laugh at themselves, laugh at their mistakes, laugh at misfortune, and to roll with the ups and downs of life. Put even more simply, when you are no longer a victim, you feel comfortable in your own skin. You can then really laugh and have fun.

23

Laughter of Joy

A friend had a granddaughter with terrible lung disease that was steadily progressing. It was incurable. Her lung capacity was steadily decreasing. My friend asked prayers for her granddaughter from everyone she knew. Many prayed intensely for her. The little girl's condition was clearly terminal. Unless she had a lung transplant she would die. Her lungs had diminished to one-third normal capacity, and her blood oxygen was dangerously low. Then the miracle happened.

A sixteen year-old boy died in a tragic car accident and his parents gave his organs to five other people so that they would live and flourish. The little granddaughter got both his lungs. It took some time for her tissue rejection medications to be fine-tuned, but today she is a thriving teenager with over 93% normal lung function.

Her family wanted to contact the donor family to personally thank them for saving their daughter's life. It took the donor family of the young man time to deal with their grief before they allowed the girl's family to correspond with them. The donor family described their son's wonderful laughter.

The girl's parents told them this story. "As her new lungs began to function better, our daughter began to laugh. She sounded different. She had never laughed this way before. Her tone of voice had changed. It was a different voice."

Their daughter's joyous laughter was not only of their daughter, but also of the young man whose lungs were giving her new life.

The girl's family did not tell the donor family the rest of the story. Their daughter had told them that every night the spirit of the young man came and visited her and wished her good night. He was telling her how happy he was that she was living and enjoying life through the gift of his lungs.

In a similar way, to fully flourish in recovery, fun and laughter are essential.

Try living with the "laughter of joy."

24

Success is the Best Solution – How Full of Fun and Laughter is That?

Abraham Lincoln ran many times for public office and he was often defeated, but he kept striving for success. He had two businesses failures, lost eight elections, and had a nervous breakdown. He kept on getting up from every defeat and became the sixteenth President of the United States.

When my wife of thirty years left me, in part for a well-paying job, and moved to Kansas City, it was devastating. Shortly, I was promoted from Lieutenant Colonel to Colonel in the 35th Infantry Division at Fort Leavenworth. Then I was recruited by the famous Menninger psychiatric hospital as an addiction therapist. Eventually I became the senior addiction therapist.

The old saying, "Success is the best revenge" can become true in recovery, but not with a revengeful attitude. Revenge poisons a person and has no place in full recovery. I found that I had to forgive myself for the negative things I had done in the marriage, and I had to forgive her for the negative things she had done. I focused on the soldiers I was helping; I focused on the patients I was treating; and I focused on the students that I was teaching in the nearby university. I did not lose my focus.

To the best of my ability, I kept going to Al-Anon, to worship services, to Alcoholics Anonymous, and continued to volunteer in various helping organizations.

Success is the best outcome, not the best revenge.

25

Jumping into Mud Puddles
Having Fun and Laughter
with Other Children

Recovery means that we humble ourselves like children and allow ourselves to have genuine, messy, fun with other people, just as a child in a new playground automatically runs and plays with other children.

Erin MacPherson tells a wonderful story in *Daily Guideposts* (2014, pg 261) about how she saw her children "taking flying leaps off the porch, into a giant mud puddle. I wanted to call them inside before I ended up spending hours scrubbing mud-splattered clothes and drying out soaked shoes, but then I saw those big, wonder-filled smiles and forgot all about things like bleach and muddy footprints tracked across clean floors."

Erin then made a decision to join the fun and laughter of her children. She herself jumped off the edge of the porch, into the mud puddle and, for half an hour, played and splashed with them in the mud. At first her children were shocked, but then they became delighted and joined right in.

In recovery we will miss joys and laughter like this unless, in many different ways, and in many different situations, we make a conscious decision to have fun and to laugh, and to get dirty in life with others.

Humbling ourselves like a child to have fun and laughter is a good idea.

26

Playfulness and Elephants and Fun and Laughter and Love

Charles LaFond lived in an elephant camp in Thailand. "When I took my elephant to the river to wash," he has said, "she loved to spray me with water from her trunk." The elephant was having fun. "When I scrubbed her back she made the elephant equivalent of a purr."

Charles developed a friendship with his elephant. "She would reach out, place her trunk on my forehead, and sigh. This always made me cry a bit."

This was Charles' first step in learning to trust the world and to like himself, just as his elephant loved him.

"One day I had trouble climbing onto my elephant's back for the day's ride. So she picked me up, with her trunk between my legs, and tossed me onto her forehead. She loved me. From that day on she always lifted me up onto her head."

Charles' elephant became a symbol to him of a loving higher power. Charles gradually rejoined the human race, finding inner healing and recovery through fun and laughter with a wonderful, playful elephant.

(Source: *Meeting God Day by Day,* 2014, pg 176).

27

Yoga and Fun and Laughter in Recovery

A few years ago, I joined Ginnie Schirmer's yoga class at Evangel United Methodist Church. As a teen I had learned a few yoga poses and practiced them after reading a beginners' book. Doing more complex yoga stances, as a senior adult in a group, revealed to me an entirely different world.

The first thing I had to relearn was balance. All I could do was laugh at myself as I staggered from front to back and from left to right. It takes a surprisingly large amount of strength and agility to stand still on one foot for any length of time. Others in the class also laughed at their own difficulties. Even Ginnie herself, as an accomplished student of yoga for many years, sometimes shared self-deprecating humor at her own yoga struggles.

Again, taking one's self too seriously is so foundational to recovery, re-learning how to have fun. The first time I did "downward facing dog" it was not much fun. Muscles and ligaments I never knew I had, all simultaneously began to talk to me, but I stuck it out.

It became more fun over time. Ginnie would gently guide us through each movement with her sensitive sense of humor. Her frequent admonition was, "Don't hurt yourself. If you can't do this movement, don't force it. Just try to increase your range of motion a little bit at a time."

What great recovery advice as well. Don't force your recovery, just do it a tiny step at a time. Ginnie's kindness and relaxed sense of humor allowed those of us in the class to begin to joke about our pain, to laugh at how clumsy we were, and not to take ourselves so seriously.

I have worked out for more than five decades, surfing, playing football, basketball, tennis, fighting forest fires for four years, and then trying to stay in top physical shape for 30 years in the United States Army, and I am still amazed at how tired I am after a strenuous yoga class.

The pain is worth the gain because my balance is so much better now, and I am so much more flexible. I feel much more at home in my own skin.

Balance, flexibility, laughter, fun, and feeling at home in my own skin, what better mottos for recovery can there possibly be?

28

Humor that Puts Down Others is Not Fun and Laughter - It Simply Hurts

The last live comedy show I attended in the big city taught me that passive-aggressive humor that puts down other people and harms the feelings of other people is not really humor. It is cruelty.

I felt so bad for the young man from Arkansas, sitting in the front row of the last comedy club I visited. Once the comedian learned that the young man was from the south, the comedian would not let him go, but regaled him again and again with funny but cruel discriminatory Arkansas jokes, to the point where I simply got up, walked out of the club, and left, never to go to a comedy club again, for the rest of my life.

The humor was quite funny, but it was humor that made the young man feel put down, embarrassed, and uneasy. I felt this was not something a recovering person should practice or participate in.

On a recent clean-and-sober canoe trip, I warned everyone that, if they slept near me, they needed to be able to sleep through a thunderstorm because I snored so loudly. They laughed briefly and went on their way. After we had canoed most of the day, cooked dinner over the campfire, cleaned up, and gone to our tents, my companions had temporarily forgotten my snore warning. I knew everyone was in for a snore-fest because I was so exhausted.

The next morning breakfast banter was rife with Cobb snoring stories. I had to make a decision. Would I allow myself to be hurt and embarrassed because these stories were basically

49

true, or should I join in their laughter? I realized the best thing to do was to egg them on, telling even more stories about my snoring disability than they could tell, and simply laughing with them.

The dark side of my human nature was to be tempted to talk down to them about their own snoring, their difficulties canoeing, their personality flaws, etc. but that would be retaliation, and not fun and laughter. Laughing at myself and refusing to tell hurtful but funny stories about them was the simply not the recovery way to go, so I had fun and laughter at my own expense.

Of course the truth did hurt a little, but I had a good time and not at the expense of my friends.

29

Fun and Laughter
at a Regional Medical Center

I was asked to do a workshop at a regional medical center. I told them I was writing a book on fun and laughter, and asked permission to speak on this subject. I began the workshop by telling several self-depreciating stories about my own behaviors that were funny and therapeutic. Then I divided them into small groups. I asked them to tell humorous stories about their experiences working in the medical center or in their own personal lives. I asked them not to tell stories that put other people down.

Immediately the large room began developing into a cacophony of laughter. They never thought they would have so much fun in a mandatory hospital workshop.

Then I asked each group to select the funniest story told in that group and to select a spokesperson to tell it. As the workshop developed and they told their hilarious stories, a sense of camaraderie and friendship began enveloping the room.

What a great way to live and to interact with other human beings.

30

Fun and Laughter in Helping Others

I went to jail again. Every Tuesday a friend and I bring Narcotics Anonymous meetings to the local jail. Unlike many of the inmates, I was never caught. I did my questionable deeds alone, unseen by anyone else because I had seen so many of my friends have their "so-called" friends "roll-over" on them when they were arrested so they could get off most of their charges. Jesus taught that we should visit people who were sick or who were in jail, so I was also obeying his command in visiting and trying to help inmates.

I am constantly amazed listening to civilians discuss the Hebrew Scriptures and the Christian Scriptures. They too often act as if the Ten Commandments and the teachings of Jesus were take-it-or-leave-it *suggestions*. Thirty years in the United States Army have caused me to recognize commands. Moses teachings and Jesus' teachings are a lot more than just gentle suggestions, they are *serious commands*. Virtually every command of Moses and Jesus are very healing and helpful to the person obeying them when they are followed. Like all commands, often I don't want to follow them, but the benefits of trying to follow them (no one but no one follows every Biblical teaching perfectly) bring incredible benefits, lead to higher self-esteem, and ultimately take us down the road of fun and laughter and peace.

What fun and joy to be a part of helping fellow human beings who originally were in such emotional pain, often abandoned by family and "friends" because of their incarceration. What fun and laughter to see young men get treated for mental health disorders and substance abuse and stop ruining their bodies and harming their communities. What fun and laughter to see these men find a productive jobs and meaning and purpose in life.

31

Fear of a Barracuda Turns
into Fun and Laughter

I tried to encourage soldiers to take advantage of free "space available" flights with the United States Air Force. On Space-A flight, I took two sergeants with me to have fun with the Air Force Band, as they played in Saint Croix and then in St. Thomas in the Virgin Islands.

The female sergeant found a handsome sergeant in the band and began to hang out with him in St. Croix. The male sergeant began to taste all of the Caribbean rum drinks he could get his hands on. I purchased a snorkel and a facemask, and went diving near the concrete foundation footings of a large hotel that stretched far out into the bay.

I dove underwater and followed small schools of fish into deeper water when, suddenly, there was very large barracuda with huge, ferocious teeth inches away from my facemask.

I began swimming backward underwater, keeping my eyes on this frightening monster. When I swam backward through a school of fish, and they scattered in all directions, I thought I was being attacked by a barracuda behind me, but then I saw the small fish scattering away from me. The large barracuda did not chase me, but stayed close to the concrete foundation, near the deep water.

The next day, the band flew in their military transport plane from St. Croix to St. Thomas, and I was sitting next to a big African American Air Force sergeant who was in the band. I told him this story. He began to laugh.

"Sir, that barracuda is named Sam. He never hurts anyone. He just hangs out by that foundation to wait for people to scare fish to him."

"Sergeant," I replied, "why couldn't you have told me that before I went snorkeling?" I gave that sergeant my best barracuda laugh. Then we both laughed at my expense.

Often in life things that first appear dangerous and frightening later prove to be nothing. Fun and laughter at our own expense, and daily effort not to take ourselves too seriously, are the secrets of a happy recovery from mental illness, substance use disorders, and physical illness.

32

Fulfillment and Deep Joy
When You Decide to Do the Right Thing

Juan Gonzalez was an anthropologist who worked with several Native American tribes in a country in South America. In doing his duties, years ago he worked under mandated national laws. Several of these regulations bothered him. He began to realize several specific injustices that were being done to Native Americans in that nation. As time went on, he found more unjust policies and discriminatory laws. It became such an ethical issue to him that he could no longer remain silent about so many policies that treated the Native peoples as second class citizens.

He protested. He advocated change. Change did not occur. His protests were unfruitful. He resigned his secure job. He was burned out, fighting the system.

Juan left direct anthropology work with the native peoples in that nation, and began his own business. Over time he developed a reputation doing outstanding, quality work. The Native peoples, whom he had been helping, also began to thrive financially. They developed a tourism niche and other industries. They remembered Juan and how he had advocated for them. He had skills they needed. They began to work with him in business ventures. Juan had genuinely cared for these Native peoples.

What fulfillment and joy to now work with the native peoples he had previously tried to protect. He had done the right thing. He had kept his integrity and his ethics.

Money cannot buy integrity. Money cannot purchase the fulfillment that Juan Gonzalez now experiences working as a business partner with these same tribes.

There are few things that can satisfy as deeply as this. Ethics is a huge part of having fun and laughter in recovery.

33

Hebrew Insights into Fun and Laughter

Laughter often can arise from deep despair. Abraham and Sarah tried to have a child all their lives. They had given up and had accepted a childless old age. Then three tired, hungry, strangers appeared. Abraham welcomed them, prepared food for them, and aided them according to the social code of that time in the Middle East. The Hebrew Scriptures teach that Abraham and Sarah did not realize they were hosting three angels.

When the men were preparing to leave, their leader told Abraham, "At this same time next year you will have a son."

Abraham did not believe it.

Sarah had her ear to the tent and was listening to every word, as was also the custom of women in nomadic tribes. When the stranger uttered these words, she laughed. She laughed so loud that the man heard her. When one of the men said he heard her laugh, she lied. "I did not laugh," she said.

"Yes you did," said the man. "I heard you laugh."

One year later, as the angel of God has prophesied, Sarah gave birth to a baby boy. They named him Isaac which means "He laughs." Abraham and Sarah's old age was full of laughter as their only son grew up.

Today Isaac is the fourteenth most common male name in Australia, the twenty-seventh most common name for boys in Canada, and the thirty-first most common name for boys in the United States.

Many people do not know the details of ancient Hebrew history, or this story about laughter in the lives of Abraham and Sarah, in Genesis 17.

There is deep wisdom in Sarah and Isaac's life-stories. When good things happen, laugh. Name the laughter, point it out. Remember that moment of laughter for the rest of your life and relish it.

There are also deep insights in Sarah's words, "God has blessed me with laughter and all who get the good news will laugh with me."

Share your laughter with your friends and with all who hear your good news. What good mental health, to be openly thankful to God for every good thing and to make it a regular habit to laugh with your friends and neighbors.

34

Praise and Thank You, Good Mental Hygiene from the 100th Psalm

*O*n your feet now—applaud God! Bring a gift of laughter, sing yourselves into his presence. Know this: God is God, and God, God. He made us; we didn't make him. We are his people, his well-tended sheep. Enter with the password: "Thank You!" Make yourselves at home, talking praise. Thank him. Worship him. For God is sheer beauty, all-generous in love, loyal always and ever. The Message Bible, Psalm 100:1-5

"Bring a gift of laughter." Hundreds of years after the lives of Abraham and Sarah, the Psalms began to be written during the time of David. The word "Psalm" is the source of the English word, "Song". The Book of Psalms is, literally, a song book. It was a hymnal for the Jewish people as they worshipped in the temple in Jerusalem, and has continued to be their hymnal throughout all of their glorious and often difficult history.

It encapsulates every emotion known to humankind showering us with an entire rainbow of emotions: from anger to peace, and from sorrow to laughter, and from Lamentations to praise. Psalm 22:3 teaches that "God inhabits the praises of his people." The 100th Psalm goes even further.

It encourages people to "applaud" God, to "talk" praise, to say "thank you," and to "bring a gift of laughter" to God.

Laughter is a gift we bring to God.

35

Another Gift of the Holy Spirit, Laughter

In Chile, South America, the Chilean Christians in the Methodist Pentecostal Church have added another gift of the Holy Spirit to the twelve gifts that Paul wrote about in I Corinthians. It is "the gift of laughter".

Laughter is, indeed, a gift. Laughter is not only a gift to God, it is not only a gift we give to others, it is one of the most precious gifts we can give to ourselves. It is a gift from the heart of the Spirit of God.

Laughter is a gift in a multitude of ways. Give yourself permission to laugh.

36

The Good Shepherd, a Lost Sheep, Meth, and Again the Shepherd Appears

The Good Shepherd was certainly watching out for Frank. He had been attending Biola University, a private Christian University in La Mirada, California, when he was seduced by both meth-amphetamines and a beautiful young woman who used meth.

He moved from California to Kansas. Through an interesting twist of circumstances we met. "What do you do?" he demanded.

I told him I was the Clinical Director of Hope Help Health and that my clinic helped persons with alcohol and drug use disorders, and also family members and the mental health disorders around alcohol and drugs.

"I'm a meth addict," Frank stated.

It was then that I realized his gruff questions were because days of using meth had made him paranoid, a common meth addict feature. I told Frank I was going to attend a Narcotics Anonymous meeting and that I would be glad to pick him up and take him with me. His paranoia kicked in again,

"Will there be police there?"

I told him there were no police there.

When the time for the meeting arrived, I decided to drive my old farm pickup truck, hoping it would lower his anxiety. He stayed for the entire meeting in spite of his severe meth-induced anxiety. I encourage him to attend NA again, but he did not show up for two years.

His amphetamine (speed, crank, and stimulant) addiction had gotten so bad that his wife had kicked him out of his home. She had gotten a restraining order, and he had been involved in an angry altercation with police. He was charged and thrown into jail.

I frequently attend a Saturday evening Spanish-speaking worship service at Evangel United Methodist Church in Holton, Kansas. When I walked in the door, Hector and Sheri Sanchez told me there was someone I needed to speak with. They introduced me to Frank. Frank recognized me from the phone call two years ago.

Hector had just prayed with Frank and now Frank told me he was now willing to go to NA or AA meetings. I gave him the day and time and location of the next meeting. Frank was there waiting. He went to other meetings.

In the next few days, his wife dropped the restraining order, the police lowered his charges from a felony to a misdemeanor, and he was placed on probation for one year. Frank began to realize that God was doing for him what he could not do for himself.

Recently Frank and his wife attended one of my meetings. Frank and Jane (not their real names) were laughing and having a good time at the meeting. At that meeting, Frank celebrated thirty days of clean time from meth. Everyone applauded his achievement. The lost sheep was returning to the fold of clean and sober living. If Frank continues to stay clean and sober, and close to the Good Shepherd the rest of his life, more healthy fun and laughter awaits him for the rest of his life. Due to past charges from the local police, Frank and his wife moved to another community. A very important part of helping other persons find recovery is to know that you have done the best job with them as you could do, but that the major part of their own recovery us up to them and them alone.

The best part of this true story is that I had just as much fun and laughter watching his recovery as did Frank and Jane.

Watching Frank change, going to meetings, and seeing their marriage strengthen, was awesome.

Fun and laughter in recovery are like ripples on a pond when a rock is thrown into still water. The fun and laughter radiates to everyone nearby, blessing them and strengthening them in their own spiritual journey of recovery.

37

A Teen Begins to Find Direction
and Meaning and Purpose

The young lady described her anxiety disorder, which she had inherited from her father. She told, in detail, the medications she was on, her precise dosages, and the medications and dosages her father took. She described, in surprising detail, how her anxiety issues and her depression issues were both similar and yet different from, those of her father.

I was amazed at the therapeutic insights this young teen had. She discussed how her social worker was able to prescribe psychotropic medications, and how her physician was also involved in her treatment and her father's pain management treatment. I asked her what goals she had for her life.

She said, "None."

I told her that I had never heard a person her age be so alert and knowledgeable about mental health issues and psychotropic medicine issues, and about pain medication issues. I encouraged her to talk with her social worker about a possible goal of becoming a social worker herself. It was not by chance that the regional mental health center in that area of the state was at that moment signing up everyday citizens for training in a course called "Mental Health First Aid". The timing of this event was unmistakable.

Later, the teen told me, with a giant smile, that she had signed up and was planning on taking this course. Regardless of whether she was able to attend it or not, it was fun to watch her go from being without purpose in life and to begin to think about a possible goal for her life.

As she talked about such a career, her eyes shined with excitement and purpose.

What fun to see this transformation take place right before my eyes. It was fun beyond joy, and laughter beyond words.

38

Love and Forgiveness and Paying It Forward Brings True Fun and Laughter

It had been a difficult summer and fall. My 96 year-old mother had gone to the hospital four times in four months for dehydration. She was noticeably weaker after each hospitalization. She had been in a good nursing home, but she was not getting quality care because of several health issues, so I had to move her to a smaller, more individually focused, facility near my home.

After months of working with her, the eighty mile round trips were exhausting me physically and emotionally. I knew I needed to take care of myself, so when mom was settled in her new suite, I attended a two and a half day retreat at King Solomon Christian Camp in Solomon, Kansas, which was one hundred miles away.

The lead speaker was a semi-retired pastor who emanated great wisdom.

"When I was young," he said, "I felt that I had to be right all of the time, but now I have learned that I needed to let some of that go and just focus on loving people and forgiving people."

It was so refreshing, because he was articulating what I was beginning to realize on my own spiritual journey.

39

The $100 Tip to the Right Person at the Right Time

On the way home from Solomon, I called my wife Kathleen and asked her to lunch at McFarland's Restaurant in the state capitol. Walt McFarland's grandfather had founded this restaurant in 1933 and for a quarter of a century it had served excellent food, had fast service, all at a reasonable price.

As we were paying our bill, Walt told us what had recently happened in his business. "One of my waitresses told me that she did not have enough money for her car insurance and she was worried about it. Later that day a young man and his wife and their two children came in for a meal. Their bill was about thirty eight dollars and he charged it on his credit card. Then I noticed that he had left a large tip. I thought he had made a mistake because the tip was for one hundred dollars. When I mentioned it to him, he replied, 'No, I did not make a mistake. Give it to our waitress. I want to pay it forward'."

Walt said, "When I gave the hundred dollar tip to my waitress at the end of the day, she began to cry. One hundred dollars was exactly the amount she needed to pay, in full, for her car insurance."

I told Walt that this entire event was a "God Thing" direct from a loving Creator.

"I know it was," he said. "When I saw it all happen, it made the hair on the back of my neck stand up."

I told him that just hearing him tell this story brought tears to my eyes. What joy and fun and laughter, and life and light, that young man brought to the waitress and to everyone who hears this story.

What joy and blessing to that young man's own life and heart.

When we have God guide our lives, as this young man did that day, it brings heaven down to earth. It is love with hands and feet. It makes a person want to go out and do likewise.

After months of seeing mom go in and out of the hospital, and get weaker each time, I was given new hope and new joy.

I needed Walt's story right then.

40

Nights of Crying Your Eyes Out Give Way to Days of Laughter

K ing David, greatest of the Jewish kings, was the focus of several assassination attempts by the first Jewish king, Saul. For years, Saul pursued David though-out Israel, Philistia, and the Negev wilderness.

The first fifty Psalms in the Hebrew Scriptures are written by David. In Psalm 30:3-5, in *The Message* translation, he expresses the full range of human emotions, from sobs to laughter. David danced with joy when the Ark of the Covenant was brought to Jerusalem. People made fun of him, including his wife, but he did not let other people keep him from joy and laughter.

Since fun and laughter are decisions as well as emotions, we are wise if we give ourselves permission to "cry our eyes out" so that we, like David, can also have "days of laughter".

–

God, you pulled me out of the grave, gave me another chance at life when I was down-and-out. All you saints sing your hearts out to God! Thank him to his face! He gets angry once in a while, but across a lifetime there is only love. The nights of crying our eyes out give way to days of laughter.

41

Subtle Humor of the Boy, Jesus of Nazareth

Jesus of Nazareth was a descendent of King David. Jesus' life shows us what might be called a "mature" sense of fun and laughter.

Jesus was 12 years old and stayed behind in Jerusalem while his parents walked back to Nazareth with other families. When Mary and Joseph could not find him, they went back to Jerusalem. They found him asking deep questions of the scribes and pharoses in the Temple. When his parents reprimanded him for not telling them where he was, he replied, "Didn't you know I had to be in my Father's house?" (Luke 2:41-52)

There is subtle humor in his reply.

Then Jesus went home and was obedient to his parents.

42

The Direct Humor of the Rabbi, Jesus of Nazareth

Two brothers, James the son of Zebedee and John his brother, became Jesus' disciples. When a Samaritan village would not accept Jesus, James and John asked if they should do exactly the same thing Elijah did in 2 Kings 1:10 when he called down fire and burned up two companies of soldiers that came to arrest him.

This may be due to the fact that some of the Jews in Israel thought Jesus might well be the reincarnation of the prophet Elijah.

"Jesus," James and John asked, "Do you want us to call down fire from heaven to destroy them?" (Luke 9:54)

I am certain that Jesus smiled as he explained to them that he was sent to earth to help and save people, not to destroy them. I believe this is why, in Mark 3:17, Jesus began calling James and John, "Sons of Thunder". They wanted thunder and fire and lightning from heaven to destroy people like Elijah, one the greatest Hebrew prophets, had done to the false prophets of Baal, on Mount Carmel.

Jesus must have quietly laughed at the misguided impetuosity of James and John as he explained to them how his mission on earth was different from Elijah's mission.

His "Sons of Thunder" comment now shows that his humor that is no longer subtle. It is very direct.

Finally, in John 15:11-15, Jesus even more clearly explains his understanding of fun and laughter and joy: "I've told you these things for a purpose: that my joy might be your joy, and your joy might be fully mature."

Jesus did not have a shallow understanding of fun and laughter. Jesus said that he was sent here to bring a deep sense of mature joy, fun, and laughter to his followers. In this passage he uses the words, "fully mature" to explain his sense of joy. We then begin to understand that Jesus' concept of fun and laughter was not a shallow thing at all, but rather consisted of experiencing a mature, profound joy of the deepest kind.

(When I directly asked Dr. Amy Levine, University Professor of New Testament and Jewish Studies at Vanderbilt University about this aspect of Jesus she said she did not believe this was a manifestation humor, but she also had no explanation as to why in the first Gospel of Mark Jesus called them "Sons of Thunder." It is clear to me that in several other passages of the four Gospels Jesus did indeed have a British type of dry humor.)

43

Native Americans and Laughter

"Laughter—that is something very sacred, especially for us Indians." John (Fire) Lame Deer, Rose Bud Lakota Sioux Nation.

"Laughter is mental. Laughter is emotional, laughter is physical, and laughter is spiritual. Laughter helps us find balance," says Terry Crossbear, a Hunkpapa Lakota (Standing Rock Sioux), on his father's side.

It was out of the Hunkpapa Lakota Nation the great prophet and leader, Sitting Bull, came. Terry is also from the Prairie Band Pottawatomie Nation, on his mother's side.

Terry shared these Native American words about laughter with me and gave me permission to publish them. "If we get too angry, laughter will turn that emotion in a balanced direction. If we have a mental picture of someone who is too strong, laughter will ease the tension. If the body is stressed, laughter will release natural relaxants into our muscles and our nervous system. Laughter often changes our attitude. We need to lighten up and laugh more. Great Spirit, teach me to laugh."

44

Laughter when another Beer is No Longer the Most Important Thing

A wise man came to me a few years ago. He was unusually wise for a person in his situation. He had a good job. He had exceptional children and a beautiful wife. He enjoyed work and loved his children and his wife, but he realized he had a problem with beer. He was wise because he knew that if he did not deal with his increasing need for alcohol he would eventually lose what he loved.

We talked several times. Eventually I asked him what time of the day he struggled most with wanting to drink excessive amounts of beer. He said it was most often in the evening, at the end of the day, when his children were in bed, and when he and his wife were just about ready to go to sleep.

At the moment he said this, a question arose in my mind. I have never asked another person this question in my entire life, but I knew this question was for him: "If your wife had just gotten in bed, and you were just about ready to get in bed yourself, in the past have you chosen to make love to your wife, or to have another beer?"

The question startled him and then he wisely gave me his honest answer. "In the past, I have decided to have just one more beer."

His answer made him realize just how much alcohol was taking over his life, and, of course, I advised him that in the future he make just the opposite decision. We candidly discussed how his repeated behavior showed beyond any doubt that having another beer was more important than making love with his wife.

A couple of weeks later, I asked him how he was doing. He said that he had taken my advice and cut out the beer and was paying more attention to his wife. I asked him if his wife had made any comments to him about this. My wise friend laughed and said, "She asked me if I had gone to my doctor and had gotten some medicine to help me."

We laughed together. What fun and laughter in recovery, to be able to laugh with my friend about the beginning of his early walk away from the life-threatening disease of alcoholism.

This is some of the best fun and laughter of all.

45

Being Part of a Tribe

I attend a wonderful Alcoholics Anonymous meeting that meets in the basement of a Catholic Church. One of the jokes in AA is that "Catholics get sober in the basements of Protestant churches." This "home meeting" is just the opposite. Protestants get sober in the basement of a Catholic church.

One evening, a friend in the group said something that helped me understand why I had decided to make this group my "home meeting". He said that when he had been drinking, he was a loner. He always drank alone. He was close to no one and he had no close friends. This is too often a typical profile of many men and women who are alcoholics.

"This meeting is my tribe," he said. "I have needed a tribe, a place to belong, for a long time. I am so grateful for this meeting."

Persons with alcohol, drug, or mental health issues, or physical health issues, are often isolated and alone. They may sometimes be near people, but they have few, close, intimate friendships with another human being. They have no one to whom they can share their deepest emotions and thoughts in a safe place. Support groups, close family groups, life-long friendships, spiritual groups, or civic service groups can help fulfill this need.

I have never laughed more than I have in my home AA group. I have never had more fun and laughter there, because I have never had more emotional pain and sorrow there either.

Fun and laugher in recovery means you allow yourself to feel the entire spectrum of normal human emotions with others, on a regular basis.

When you fully laugh, you also automatically give yourself permission to fully cry.

Join some type of tribe.

46

How the Russian Language Shows an Important Thing about Laughter

To survive the long Russian winters, people in Russian villages all have to help each other on a daily basis. "You are out of potatoes? Here are some of mine. Your baby needs milk, here. I just milked my goat this morning."

Human beings cooperate on a higher level than any other living things on our planet. The Russian language itself reflects this need to interact and to help each other.

There are very few words and concepts in Slavic languages that talk about the need for a rugged individualism that western civilization tends to promote. Rather the Russian language emphasizes cooperation, common goals, and common needs.

Everyone in the middle of an artic Russian winter, knows they need help. This is perhaps why the Russian soul is often almost Latin with its emotional and embracing style.

47

The Fun and Laughter of Seeing Babushkas at work in Russia and Slavic Nations

There are *Babushkas* in every single Slavic nation. *Babushkas* are like little grandmothers. Even if they have never seen your face, a *Babushka* will go up to you and say things like, "It is cold outside. Go back inside and put on your coat." They will walk up to a General or a Russian Prime Minister and say, "Your tie is crooked" or "Your zipper is undone", without a minutes hesitation.

Babushkas are not only accepted in Slavic societies, they are loved and appreciated. Everyone needs a friendly, helpful grandmother. A *Babushka* embraces you and affirms you, and corrects you, even if you are a total stranger. She will smile the smile only a loving grandmother can give. She makes you smile and laugh to yourself.

On a cold Russian winter day, one always uses a bit of Slavic fun and laughter. Might today be the perfect day to begin a career of being a *Babushka* to others right now?

48

Post-Traumatic Stress Disorder (PTSD) and the Need for Fun and Laughter

Trauma is a serious business. Trauma also has a lot of depression. Many soldiers, police officers, emergency room personnel, and others have already had quite a bit of trauma before the final traumatic events that put them over the edge, into a more full-blown PTSD.

PTSD has a long incubation life, and it takes as many years to treat as it did to create it. People with trauma, and with depression, tend not to have fun and laughter, even though they need them both desperately. It takes discipline to attend PTSD groups, to go to individual therapy, and to be humble enough to know that some psychotropic medicines may be needed for a more full recovery.

Some psychologists postulate that it may be four to six years for a person to even begin the process of walking away from PTSD. Like the loss of a loved one, or the loss of a marriage, one never fully recovers, but, nonetheless, recovery is possible.

The first thing to do is to talk about the trauma in enough detail that it gets solidly articulated into words. Unarticulated trauma does not work because the left brain needs concrete words to be able to help it figure out trauma issues logically. Secrets keep a person sick and the more secrets a person has, the sicker they are. A safe place to disclose secrets is needed.

A friend, from a Special Forces unit, whose platoon was able to massacre an entire battalion of Viet Cong soldiers on a top secret military mission, began to recover only when he began to tell the details of that battle. He had been sworn by National

Security to absolute secrecy about their mission. For several years the burden of holding that secret in was, literally, killing him.

What a joy to see the tension ease from his face as he told his story. He began to relax.

It will be a long journey back to a more normal life, but now my friend is gradually learning how to have more of a capacity for fun and laughter in his recovery.

49

Brett Favre in Retirement Re-learns Fun and Laughter in Recovery

B rett says that the hardest thing about leaving National Football League and the Green Bay Packers was the loneliness and loss of the comradeship of being with other team members. He did not know what to do. It was traumatic for him to no longer be on the field with his NFL friends and colleagues. He decided to offer his services as an unpaid coach for his local high school football team.

"I did not want to be the head coach. I just wanted to be one of the coaches," he said. Teaching young players how the play the game he loved, and eventually being able to help that high school team to a state championship, have given Brett much needed meaning and purpose in life.

There is an old Midwestern saying: "A man who keeps to himself makes a mighty small package." Brett realized he needed other people. He had a skill that he could teach others. He found others willing, and wanting to have him teach them. Brett now has young men from all over his region who can proudly say, "My coach was Brett Favre." Brett can now proudly say, "I helped teach him to play ball and look how well he is doing now."

Brett Favre's life now has a reservoir of fun and laughter in recovery as he helps others.

50

I Have Not Heard My Son
Laugh Like That in a Long Time

My friend was so concerned about her son. He would get a good job, drink too much alcohol, and because of his alcohol problem, lose that job. He would get in a positive relationship, drink too much alcohol, and lose that relationship. This went on for twenty years.

My friend began to attend Al-Anon. She started focusing on herself and stopped focusing on her alcoholic son. She stopped rescuing him. She started to realize that she could not change him and whenever she rescued him, it just enabled him to drink that much longer. She took her hands off of his life and started to work the 12 Steps of AA herself.

With this history in mind, it was so much fun to hear her most recent story.

"My son finally got this well-paying job in a factory. He is a hard worker and, when he finished at his work station, he would go to another part of the factory where they needed help. The other worker was a Native American man from Guatemala who was about 5'2", squat, and built like a fire plug. He needed help lifting a heavy box. My son is 6'4" and, as he helped lift the box, he soon realized that their size difference made him impossible to help lift that box. At that same moment the Guatemalan worker said, 'You too tall. You too tall.' My son called me on the phone and told me this story. He laughed as he repeated, 'You too tall. You too tall.' It has been a long time since I have heard him laugh like that."

My friend instinctively realized that her son had stopped drinking and was in recovery because of his wholehearted laughter.

People in recovery can have fun and laughter even in workplaces in situations like this.

51

Fun and Laughter at 92 Years of Age

Jacques Casparian, MD, the best dermatologist I have ever had, told me an interesting story about a 92 year-old patient. After Dr. Casparian examined him, he asked his secret to having such healthy skin, such vibrant health, and such an ageless appearance.

The man described how he exercised regularly, how he ate only healthful foods, and other details of how well he took care of himself. At the end, he gave one more detail. "I also was a boxer. Once I boxed six rounds with Dempsey."

Dr. Casparian was immediately perplexed and began thinking, *How could he box against Dempsey? He was a heavyweight boxer and much bigger.*

Jack Dempsey had been the world heavyweight champion from 1919-1926. He was 6'1" and stocky and strong. Dempsey was from Manassa, Colorado, had initially gotten a reputation for winning fights in his small Colorado town, began boxing nationally, and then became a legend not only in the boxing world, but eventually became an American cultural hero. The 92 year-old man whom Dr. Casparian saw before him was nowhere near that tall or as stocky as a heavyweight boxer. There was no way this older gentleman could have stayed in the ring that long with Dempsey.

The patient, seeing the disbelief written all over his doctor's face, laughed and said, "The referee was named Dempsey."

What a wonderful story about taking care of yourself and retaining a healthy sense of humor far into old age. Scientifically, we know that fun and laughter changes brain chemistry in a healthy way. This new brain chemistry then is healing to the entire body.

In sharing this joke with his dermatologist, the old gentleman was subconsciously revealing one foundational reason for his healthy skin and vibrant health. He could laugh at himself and have fun. Research shows that mental health issues, addiction issues, and physical health issues, all improve when a person practices fun and laughter in recovery, otherwise, why recover?

52

There is a Special Vitamin
for Fun and Laughter in Recovery

D r. Mehmet Oz, a popular television medical doctor in the United States, has called friendship "Vitamin F." From a medical standpoint, Dr. Oz realized that people need friendship just as much as they need physical vitamins. He believes that without friends, our mental health and our physical health are hampered.

Studies of the communities in the world, where people live to over 100 years of age on a regular basis, reveal many scientific facts that support Dr. Oz's thesis. In every one of these communities, very old adults are treated with respect and have a wide circle of friends of all ages to give them unconditional support and love.

Friends also help a person to become more forgiving, more compassionate, kinder, and more patient, and all of these character strengths have been proven to improve physical, mental, and psychological health.

Close friends know all of your character flaws and still accept you. Thus, friends help us learn how to forgive ourselves, which is an important foundational basis of all good mental hygiene. We can have fun and laugher with friends.

For over 30 years, I have canoed throughout the United States and Canada with Bruce Ames. We have laughed together and struggled through difficult times together. We have canoed many different rivers together, in flood stage and in drought.

Dr. Oz is right. Friendship is indeed Vitamin F.

53

There Was No Room in the Inn for the King of the Universe

It was December. I was thinking of how Jesus' parents had found no room in the **Inn**, even though Jesus was the **King** of Creation coming into the world.

I had just finished visiting a friend after her surgery and was driving down the main street of Hiawatha, Kansas, on my way to a Chinese restaurant. A sign on the right side of the main street caught my eye because it had the words **"Inn"** and **"King."** When I read the sign I had a good laugh. It read, *"Dewdrop **Inn**, Budweiser **King** of Beers."*

It was a different kind of **Inn** and a different kind of **King.** I am sure there were friendly, kind, people in that bar that afternoon, as there are in every small town bar in Kansas, but I was thinking about worshiping another kind of king. There is no question in my mind that God has a well-developed sense of humor, and laughed along with me that afternoon on my way to the Chinese restaurant.

54

Tim Townsend's Adventures Exemplify Fun and Laughter in Recovery

It was fun watching Tim Townsend grow up in Oakland Christian Church. He went on the first church ski trip. I showed him how to snowplow so he could slow down when he went on his first ski run.

Winter Park ski area, in Colorado, has a very wide beginners' slope, but it was so steep it was almost a blue-liner or intermediate slope. Tim got off the ski lift and began to go straight down the mountain. Apparently he got going so fast, so quickly, that he thought it would be impossible to do a snow plow.

I had skied down the slope ahead of him and was watching him from outside the ski lodge with his parents, Hubert and Betty Townsend. He was gaining more and more speed. Fortunately, there were no other skiers in front of him. He was headed straight for the main ski lodge building.

We were all holding our breath and finally relaxed when, to avoid hitting the building, he fell down on purpose, at the end of his run. Tim laughed right along with us, at his first ski adventure.

In the fall of the next year, the Townsends were with us at the family ranch in Bourbon County, Kansas. We were cooking dinner over a fire outside. It was evening and the sun was going down. The ranch is in the Little Osage River Valley and our creek was full of heavy timber: oaks, hickories, ash, heavily forested.

"I'm going down the creek for a hike," he said.

There was an abandoned farm house to the south and west where, every year, a coyote raised her puppies.

I warned Tim, "It won't be long before the coyotes are out and howling as they chase rabbits."

"I will be okay," Tim said, as he walked down into the forest valley.

About fifteen minutes later, the mother coyote and her puppies began chasing a rabbit and howling and screaming as only a young coyote pack would do. They were not far from Tim and their loud cries were echoing up the valley, intensified by the creek's rocky bluff.

In a very short time, Tim came running and stood by the fire, next to us. It took several minutes for him to catch his breath. We laughed with Tim and he laughed with us as well.

We see again in Tim's stories how important it is in mental health, physical health, and in recovery from substance abuse, that we retain the ability to laugh at ourselves and, thereby, have more fun in life.

People in recovery can laugh at themselves. People not in recovery take themselves too seriously. Tim laughed.

55

Serious Joy and Laughter from a 3:00 AM Answered Prayer in Vietnam

People who passionately love or who are experiencing intense emotional and physical stress, can sometimes have wonderful psychic experiences. This true story took place during the Vietnam War.

Sally's son was serving in a military unit that was in the middle of some of the worst conflict. Sally prayed every day and night for his safety. One night, as was her usual pattern, she prayed for her son before she went to sleep.

"I woke up at three AM in the morning. I knew he was in danger. I asked God to protect him. At that exact moment, her son was playing poker with several other soldiers in Vietnam. They had come in from patrol and they were relaxing. Suddenly, he stood up.

"I didn't know why," he explained later, "but I put my cards down and walked out the door. Just as soon as I closed the door a mortar round came down and landed exactly where I was sitting. I know it was my mother's prayers at that same moment at home that helped the Good Lord protect me."

Fun and laughter in recovery is not only about boisterous laughter, but also can be about serious joy. It is fun to watch Sally talk about this and to see her son smile and laugh with her, with a thankful heart for the immediate answered prayer clear across the United States and the Pacific Ocean at three AM in the morning, Central Standard Time.

56

Real Wyoming Cowboys Can Have Fun and Laughter and So Can Others

Uncle Don and Aunt Leta Hoffman and my three cousins lived in Buffalo, Wyoming. There were several large cattle ranches surrounding Buffalo that hired a lot of cowboys. Uncle Don was an auctioneer and knew everyone.

Once, when my family was visiting, the Hoffman's told this interesting cowboy story. Remember that this story took place many years ago in the middle of the 20th Century.

When they got paid each month, many of the cowboys would go into town on the weekend. Some would have too much to drink and would start shooting out the streetlights. They would be arrested, sober up in jail, go back to their ranch, and the cycle would start over again the next payday.

Most of the townspeople and the cowboys would laugh at their behaviors. Life was slower and simpler then and it was probably one of the few exciting things going on in that small town on the vast plains below the Buffalo Range of the Rocky Mountains.

Such behavior would not be so easily tolerated in the 21st Century. It was a more innocent age. It is something we can look back upon as a history of the Wild West, but wouldn't it be fun to begin to view the questionable actions of other people in a less serious mode from time to time, and to give young men from lonely ranch work a little more leeway? No, I am not advocating that you drink too much and, please, don't shot out the streetlights.

57

Rancho Oso, Two Cowboys, a Bobcat, and a Lot of Burlap Bags

My first job was working at Rancho Oso, for Bob Jamison, in the Santa Ynez Valley, in Los Padres National Forest, when I was in seventh grade. There I heard about two Rancho Oso cowboys. One day their dog treed a bobcat in a big oak tree. They let their dog keep the bobcat up in the tree all day, until they could get off work. Then one of them said, "I think we can catch that bobcat alive. It might be worth more money alive than dead."

"How can we do that?" the other cowboy asked.

"We have a lot of burlap bags over there; we can use those."

It took them quite a while to catch that bobcat, and everyone who saw them the next few days asked, "What in the world happened to you?" because they saw the claw marks all over their arms and upper body.

"We caught a bobcat alive," they said, and would tell their story and then, at the end, they would laugh and say, "We are never going to do that again."

When we make a mistake and tackle something that is way too much for us, wouldn't it be wise to just laugh about it and not take our actions too seriously? What if we acted like those two cowboys and simply laugh and say, "I am not going to do that again."

Then we can let painful things go and get on with our lives.

58

Wild Driving, Inappropriate Seating, and Not Taking Yourself Too Seriously

A large rancher, in a black cowboy hat, shared some homespun wisdom with me as I was writing this book. His story was both pretty rough and pretty right.

"I had an Alcoholics Anonymous sponsor who was a crazy man. He gave me a lot of good advice to help me quit drinking, but the most important thing he taught me was to enjoy life, laugh, and not take myself too seriously.

"I don't like to go to AA meetings where they wear suits. Those type of people seem to take themselves far too seriously. My sponsor was a skinny old guy who walked with a limp, but he thought he was *The Man*. One time, he took me in his car to an AA meeting that was several miles away, and nearly scared me half to death. He believed that you should drive five miles per hour faster than the highest number on your speedometer. I was never so glad to get to a meeting alive in all my life. I stopping going to meetings with him and started taking my own car.

"In this particular meeting people would dress in fancy clothes. We were just wearing casual clothes. The women at that meeting would sit on one side and men would sit on the other side. We went in the door and he said, 'Follow me,' so, even though he was a little wimpy guy, I obeyed him. He had a big voice.

"He sat down on the women's side. He motioned for me to sit down right next to him. More than one man came over and told us, 'We don't think you will feel comfortable here.'

95

"He replied, 'We are perfectly comfortable.'

"After the meeting we laughed a lot about it."

"For a person to get over alcohol and drugs they need to stop taking themselves so seriously and they need to loosen up. I think that people who commit suicide are taking themselves far too seriously. If alcoholics can get in this AA program and lighten up, and not take themselves so seriously, they will find recovery."

59

The Joy of Getting Rid of a Long-Term Resentment

I had an aunt, Isola Cobb, with whom I wanted to stay in touch because she lived far out in Wyoming where I had a large extended family. I put her name and address on the church newsletter mailing list because each month I wrote a long, personal column in that newsletter. I wanted her to know what was going on in my life. After a few weeks, I got a scathing letter back from my far-away aunt that essentially said she gave to her own church and she was not going to give to my church and she didn't want to get any newsletter from my church.

Her letter stung me to the core. Money was not my intent at all. She was elderly and I simply wanted to stay in touch with her. I felt hurt, embarrassed, misunderstood, and angry. I wrote her back (this was in the days before emails) and told her that my only reason for mailing the newsletter was to stay in touch with her and to let her know what was going on in my life. I ended the letter with, "Believe me, I will immediately take you off the church mailing list."

She wrote me back a letter of apology, but I was so upset I never responded.

A few years later, when I was back in Wyoming visiting other relatives, I was told this same aunt was in the hospital, dying. I went alone to the hospital to be with her, to say goodbye and to have a prayer with her. It was in her room I realized my old resentment was still there.

Immediately I understood it was not by chance I was back in Wyoming at precisely the time she was dying.

She was only semi-conscious. I took her hand, told her I forgave her, and had a prayer with her, asking God to guide her on her journey and to bless her in the life to come. The peace that washed over me was so amazing, it felt like joy. It was joy. It was freedom. The burden of resentment had lifted from my shoulders. It was a feeling of lightness deeper than words can say. My forgiveness for her behavior had substance and strength and deep healing in it.

How can I have fun and laughter in recovery if I have resentment toward others?

60

Freed of the Ghosts of the Past
to Live with Peace Before She Died

She was a beautiful Native American lady. She began to talk about the pain of her past. When she was three years old, when her two teenage uncles had sexually abused her. When her father came home, she grabbed him by his knees, and told him what had just happened. Her father was a very tall and a very big Native American man who owned a saw mill. He was incredibly strong from moving heavy logs day after day, year after year.

As soon as he heard from his little daughter what had they had done, he told her to sit downstairs and to wait for him. He went upstairs to her two uncles. She heard banging and screaming. Then it became quiet. Her father came downstairs and told her that her uncles would never bother her again.

Her uncles disappeared. Everyone asked where they were. No one ever heard of them anymore. They vanished. No one knew. Her father said he did not know what had happened to them.

When the little girl grew up, she began to drink a lot of alcohol trying to push away the memories of her two uncles' behaviors. When her father died, she still worried about her uncles harming her, and continued to drink.

Her mother died. She raised a family and she still worried and drank. Finally, after her family was raised, she began to talk about this childhood trauma to a trusted friend. When she had finished, her friend told her that she would never have to worry about her uncles again. She asked why. Her friend said it was obvious. Her father had killed her two uncles on the same day they had harmed her.

She sat in stunned silence. She smiled. She laughed. She put her head in her hands. Then she cried as she laughed, "Oh good! They will never harm me again!"

All her life she had been deeply fearful that her predatory uncles would somehow reappear. Finally she had told this trusted friend about it. It was a terrible secret. She was now free from fear. The little, previously untreated, three year-old girl inside of her no longer had to be afraid of her two abusive uncles.

She quit drinking. She died just a few months later, after being treated, not only for her alcoholism, but was now also treated for her sexual abuse and trauma issues.

Sober, she felt the whole range of normal emotions again. She cried. She laughed. She often smiled. She was free. She died a whole person.

61

The Ghost in the Ozark Mountain Valley
or *a Good Reason Not to Drink*

John O'Malley was a hard-working Scotch-Irish immigrant. He restricted his drinking to Friday nights only, since many in the O'Malley clan had a serious history of alcohol abuse. Every Friday night, after a long week of hard work, he would get on his mule, Betsey, and ride her down a well-worn trail, into town. He had an agreement with his wife and children that he would never be home later than midnight.

Not far from his home the trail went down a steep mountain valley. After coming out of the valley, the trail was longer but easier, yet it was the Ozark Mountains after all, where no trail and no road could be absolutely straight or absolutely level. This was during the time that the United States Forest Service was purchasing mountain land for recreational purposes, but not much activity had gone on around the O'Malley homestead.

After several drinks, promptly at eleven PM, John would leave the tavern every Friday, get on Betsey, lay the reins down, and let her work her way back home, down the trail. They were almost home one night, and had gone down into the bottom of the deep valley not far from O'Malley homestead, when Betsey stopped. She refused to go forward.

John was rather groggy from downing several pints, but Betsey's sudden stop jolted him awake. No amount of urging would make Betsey go forward. The Scotch-Irish of the Ozark Mountains, similar to the Scotch-Irish of the Appalachian

Mountains, are quite superstitious. Finally, John O'Malley saw the reason for Betsey's unusual behavior.

It was very dark that night. There was no light. Clouds were even blocking out the starlight, but there it was. It was a white figure, about the size of a man, on the trail. Immediately John thought this was a "haunt" or a ghost on the trail.

At that point O'Malley became as frightened as his mule. He quickly back-tracked the very long trail back to the tavern and then had to take a circular, much longer route, home. When he finally got home, about one-thirty AM, his wife and children were all awake and out of bed, worried that, riding home drunk, some accident had happened to John and Betsey.

When they asked him, he explained he and Betsey had seen a "haunt" in the bottom of deep valley trail near their home. He said it was white, the size of a man, and Betsey could not be persuaded in any way to go past it. It had to be a ghost.

The next day, all of the tired family members slept in late. They were curious beyond measure so, even before breakfast, the whole family walked down the trail, to the bottom of the valley where Betsey and John had seen the "haunt." Then they saw it.

It was white. It was the size of a man. It was exactly as John had described it. As they got closer, they realized what it really was. It was a new United States Forest Service sign, giving trail directions.

The old Ozark mountain man who told me this tale swore up and down it was true when I was on a canoe trip there. I wish I knew the end of the story. I hope John O'Malley quit drinking for good after being scared out of his mind that dark night by that sign. I hope he was able to laugh at himself and what happened that night as he told his tall tale with other recovering alcoholics. A scare like this is, indeed, just one other good reason not to heavily drink, even on Friday nights, in a binge weekend alcoholic pattern.

62

Another Irish Story and another Reason Not to Drink Too Much Alcohol

Southeast Kansas, in the Little Osage River Valley, is a lot like the Ozark Mountains. The valleys are full of burr oaks, red oaks, post oaks, hickory trees, and tall sycamore trees. The ridges are filled with thick, tall, grass prairie. The Cobb family ranch, La Tierra de la Paz, is located in this beautiful area.

About a mile east down the Little Osage River is a peaceful side-valley which the locals call "Irish Valley" because several Irish immigrant families had moved there in the late 1800's. My nearest neighbor, Scott Northway, whose people had lived in this valley since before the Civil War, told me this story.

When someone died in Irish Valley, the custom was to prepare their body for burial, place them in a coffin in their own home, invite all the friends and neighbors over, and have a night-long Irish "wake" with food and alcohol. Then they would take the body to the cemetery.

The nearest Catholic Cemetery, from Irish Valley, was five miles east, to Mapleton, Kansas, and then a few more miles east, to Fulton, Kansas. Before reaching the cemetery, the funeral party would have to ford the river since, in those early days there were no bridges over the Little Osage River.

His friends and family at the wake propped the body of Thomas O'Shea up in his casket in his house, and drank and talked to him—and about him—all night. Before sunrise, they began the long trip to the Catholic Cemetery just west of Fulton, Kansas, for his graveside service.

They put his body in a wooden, horse-drawn wagon, and drank and talked the entire trip.

When they got to the cemetery, they turned around and found that O'Shea was not in the wagon. He and his casket were gone. The river had been higher than usual when they forded it, and they realized the casket had floated out of the wagon and had floated down river.

They quickly drove the wagon back to the ford where they had crossed the river. Several men began walking down the river in the early morning light, looking for O'Shea in his wooden casket. Finally, they found him a long way down the river. It seemed to take forever because it was very hard work, pushing him and his casket upstream, against the current, back to the wagon at the ford in the river.

O'Shea was almost late to his own graveside service because of the inattentive behavior of his inebriated family and friends.

Every time I remember this true tall tale, I experience fun and laughter.

63

Lizard Lips, Total Exhaustion, and Humor in the Middle of the Night

We were on field training exercises at Fort Riley, Kansas. We were in a jeep driven by a tall and lanky black sergeant whom everyone loved for his great sense of humor. We had been firing field artillery for several days and nights, and were exhausted.

The password to get back to our tent area was "Lizard Lips". Each word needed to be put in a separate paragraph so only that gate guards would recognize it. Any enemy listening to the long conversation would miss the two passwords because "lizard" would be separated by several sentences from "lips."

Our sergeant decided he would make those two passwords into a humorous story. Here we are, four exhausted soldiers, in full battle-rattle, crammed in an old Army jeep at three AM. All of us knew the passwords, so we were waiting for them. His story got longer and longer, and funnier and funnier. By the time he got to the passwords, all four of us in the jeep, and all the gate guards, were laughing so much our stomachs hurt.

All of this took place at three AM. We were tired beyond measure and yet we were having fun.

Life can be exhausting and difficult at times, but even then, laughter can lift us to new heights. If we act like this fine sergeant, we can lead others to fun and laughter in recovery, even in the middle of the night.

64

Fun and Laughter after an A-10 Gunship Encounter at Fort McCoy

We had been in an endless stop-and-go military convoy from Kansas City, Missouri to Fort McCoy, Wisconsin, for many long hours. When we finally got there, we joined six thousand soldiers in the field. Sixteen soldiers got hit by lighting. One young man's pelvis was crushed. We had to relieve our company commander of duty for sleep deprivation. He almost drove us over a cliff in the middle of the night.

It was a huge war game. Every night, opposition forces would attack and probe our perimeter defenses, and M-16's and machine guns would fire all night long. Even when the weapons were not firing, loud electrical generators shattered the sound all night long. It was raining much of the time. We were miserable. No one knew exactly where friendly forces were located in the "fog of battle" exercise.

After days and nights of sleeplessness, I developed an action plan. In the middle of the night, I low crawled between two machine gun nests to get away from all the noise. I found a thick forest of young pine trees. There was a foot of soft pine needles underneath them. I crawled up underneath the trees, laid down on my back, with my helmet on my head, and immediately went to sleep.

Just as the sun came, an A-10 gunship (affectionately called a "Warthog") passed a few feet over the pine trees. It fired its tank-busting Gatling guns. Each Gatling gun shell is several inches long and, when it fires, it is much louder than thunder.

At the first burst of gunfire I reflexed upright with such force that my helmet struck a low pine branch and knocked me out. When I came to I started laughing and laughing and laughing. I had low crawled into an A-10 tank-buster gunnery range.

As soon as I collected myself, I got back to our unit area and was able to crawl between the same two machine gun nests. No one noticed I had been gone.

It was several years before I shared this story. Laughing at myself, and taking myself less seriously, is a foundational feature of my own recovery. At this point in the book, are you starting to be able to laugh at yourself? What A-10 gunnery range have you crawled into lately?

65

Heat, Humidity, Cool Cave, Cold Water, and Fun and Laughter

Moments of joy can unexpectedly appear even in the most difficult of days. Fort Crowder, Missouri, at one time, had over 45,000 people during World War II. It is now a military training area and a woodland conservation area.

It was the middle of summer, and over one hundred degrees, when our Army Reserve unit was doing a field training exercise there. The humidity was almost unbearable.

I was on foot at Camp Crowder, visiting many platoons of soldiers scattered out over hundreds of acres. I got out a map and found the location of every military unit in our area. It consisted of a sloping valley with a road down each side. The troops were scattered down the south road and the north road, on the either side of the valley.

I began the dusty walk down the road on the south side of the valley, visiting each unit emplacement. When I got to the last unit on the south side, I got out the Camp Crowder map again. I saw that if I cut directly down across the valley, through the heavy timber, rather than walking the long, hot, dirt road, I would save myself a lot of walking before visiting the soldiers on the north side of the valley.

At the bottom of the valley, I was surprised to come across a swiftly flowing creek. The water was clear and cold. Turning a bend in the creek, I found an old settler cabin. Beyond the cabin

I saw the source of the water. It was flowing out of a small Ozark cave. No wonder the water was cool and clear.

I drank my fill of the water since I had no canteen and it was very hot. Then I walked into the cool of the cave and sat down. I waited until my eyes became used to the semidarkness, looked for snakes, and when I found none, laid down and immediately went to sleep. I woke up refreshed, drank more water, and then visited all the soldiers on the north side of the creek.

What surprise joy! What refreshment!

66

Covered with Ticks
and Still Having Fun and Laughter

A few years later, after two weeks of training in an area north of Camp Crowder at Camp Clark, in a similar forested east of Nevada, Missouri, every soldier in the field in our Battalion was covered with tiny "seed ticks" that are prolific in those Ozark mountain areas. I had low-crawled out of the area to bathe in a farm pond, but to no avail, I still had ticks.

In an effort to improve morale, and to provide a bit of humor to sweaty soldiers in the humid, tick-infested woods, the personnel section of our unit created a newspaper called *The Tick Haven Gazette*. It was full of useful military training information and also full of appropriate, humorous articles. We all needed a laugh in such difficult, sweaty conditions.

The last humorous thing that happened to me on that mission was as we were loading up our military vehicles to return to our home units.

We were all exhausted. A young soldier yelled out across the big parade area, "Bless me Chaplain."

I yelled back at him, "Raise your right hand."

He did.

Then I yelled back, "Bless you, my child, for I know you have sinned."

The parade ground had several soldiers nearby who heard his request. They immediately burst out into hearty laughter. We all needed more than a little bit of laughter, because it was going to take us a long time to get rid of all those tiny seed ticks.

67

Sergeant Major Fitzsimmons, a Stolen Jeep, an Explosion and Laughter

Sergeant Major (SGM) Fitzsimmons was a great guy and an excellent noncommissioned officer, so I was very disappointed when he began stealing my Army jeep on military training exercises. Every jeep had a "logbook" that was supposed to be with it at all times.

He began "borrowing" my jeep at Fort Riley so many times that finally I took the logbook into the barracks at night and slept with it in my sleeping bag. When I woke up, ate breakfast, and went out to the motor pool, my jeep was gone. I went to the motor pool sergeant.

"SGM Fitzsimmons signed it out, Sir," was the reply.

I burst into a commander's meeting and, interrupting it, I held up the logbook. I said to Lieutenant Colonel Stone, "Sir, Fitzsimmons has taken my jeep again. Here is the logbook. I am going to call the Fort Riley Military Police to arrest him."

Immediately LTC Stone replied, "Oh no. Don't do that Chaplain. I will take care of it."

Fitzsimmons never stole my jeep again.

The next year, at Fort Carson, Colorado, we were doing Field Artillery exercises in the Rocky Mountains on an 8,000 foot plateau above the Fort. It had been cold that night. Two other soldiers and I had almost run over by a jeep in the dark and found it was very hard to run while still in the Army "mummy bags", so we moved into the pine trees near the mess hall.

The sun was just coming up over the ridge when we heard a tremendous explosion. Someone had been trying to light the underwater gasoline "immersion" water heaters in a steel trashcan. I looked up to see the explosion blow the smokestack off the water heater, up into the air, like a missile.

I ran down to the soldier by the gasoline heater, who was briskly rubbing his face. It was SGM Fitzsimmons. He had been trying to warm the water up so he could have his morning shave. His mustache, his eyelids, his eyebrows, and his sideburns had all been burned off. His face was bright red. He had thrown a match down into the gasoline pouch of the heater and when the heater had not ignited, he looked down into it at the exact moment it exploded. The gas vapors had been slow to develop on that cool morning, but when they did blow up it was powerful.

I saw that Fitzsimmons was okay, minus all the hair on the front of his face, so I went back to my two friends. I told them the story of how SGM repeatedly took my jeep at Fort Riley, what had just happened to him with the mess hall water heater, and ended my story by saying, "What goes around comes around." We all had a hearty laugh at SGM Fitzsimmons' expense.

After teaching Introduction to Ethics courses at colleges and universities for years, I found that every reputable ethical system around the world, at its core has "treat others like you would like to be treated," and that what goes around, comes around.

Whenever I am unjustly treated badly, I have learned not to retaliate but simply to wait. I often think of SGM Fitzsimmons. It has been my experience that eventually, in this lifetime, those who treated me badly have almost always treated others badly. I have seen them reap the rewards of their own actions. Knowing this keeps me from having resentments. Resentment is my enemy because it keeps me from having fun and laughter in recovery.

68

Look, Sir, They Are Roasting a Dog.
It has a Tail. Its Head is Still On

Every time we left Eagle Base on a military mission I would try to bring a young soldier with us outside the steel and concrete walls, to see the real people and everyday life of Tuzla and rural Bosnia. Sometimes no one would go with me, but that day one young soldier accepted the invitation.

We would always drive past several roadside restaurants. We knew we were in a Serbian Orthodox area when we would see a hog roasting on a spit outside a restaurant. We knew were in a Bosnian, Islamic area when we saw a sheep roasting outside on a spit. Like the Jews, followers of Islam believe that pork is a forbidden food.

The young soldier with me insisted they were roasting a dog. "Look Sir, it has a tail like a dog. It still has its head on and its tongue is hanging out. It is a dog."

I explained to him they were grilling a whole sheep, but still he would not believe me. He must have been a city boy.

I stopped the military vehicles and offered to purchase a meal for every soldier and the translator with us. Most of them opted for a soda. I ordered the mutton. The restaurateur took a knife, shut the grill off, and cut several piece of meat off the sheep. Most Americans are not used to eating mutton or lamb, but I always enjoy it. The soldier tried one small bite. To this day, I think a part of that young man still thinks that I was eating a dog, even though I did my best to convince him.

113

I have fun and laughter with this memory every time I think about the dog that was really mutton.

69

Finding a Safe Place
Before Going to a Hostile Fire Zone

After 9-11 the world became a much more dangerous place for those of us in the 35th Infantry Division at Fort Leavenworth. In a few short years, soldiers from the 35th were serving in all of the major areas of conflict. One of my friends went on five different overseas rotations. The first mission of the 35th Division was to ramp up as the command and control for the SFOR 13 NATO Peacekeeping Mission at Eagle Base in Tuzla, Bosnia-Herzegovina in 2002-2003.

This took place after Desert Storm and before the second invasion of Iraq, called Enduring Freedom. I knew that for the next year of active duty we would be working stressful long hours, day after day, and that I needed a safe place to go to in my mind, when there would be chaos all around me.

In November, before the deer season began, I drove down to the family ranch on the Little Osage River in NW Bourbon County, Kansas. Before the sun went down I climbed up in my tree stand and watched the light fade away. Three does came into the meadow and peacefully grazed underneath the tree. I stayed there until it was totally dark and then quietly went back to the hunting cabin.

When we discovered a mass grave, or when we lost two soldiers, or when we had to blow up 1,200 destabilized Russian surface to air missiles, or when things got really rough, I would take a few minutes out, go back to that meadow and, in my mind, watch those deer peacefully graze.

Remembering the beauty of the scene helped restore my sanity. It brought fun and relaxation even to the middle of that busy, stressful, hostile fire zone.

70

David Albert Cobb Brings Messes and Fun and Laughter

We adopted David when he was 3 days old. Children can bring a lot of fun and laughter into your life if you allow them to do so. The doctor in Salina, Kansas, looked us both in the eyes, intuitively seeing that we were neat freaks, and said, "Remember, children make messes."

At the time, his comment surprised me, but now, years later, I look back at it and laugh. He was right, but the joy and fun and laughter David brought into our lives was well worth any "messes" David made.

71

David and the Dung Beetle

David and his mother came down to the family ranch in Bourbon County with me one summer day. For 30 years I raised cattle there with the help of my wonderful neighbor, Dale Brillhart.

I was feeding the cattle, and David and his mother were walking up the road, when they saw something move in some soft cow manure (or if you are from Kansas, cow pie). It was a dung beetle. I saw them as they both squatted down and were watching as it made a quarter inch dung ball, rolled it down the hill a short way to some softer dirt, dug a hole, and buried the ball, so the beetle could lay its eggs. The next year, when its offspring hatched, they would do the same thing.

It was a marvelous way of disposing of manure and of fertilizing the ground, that the Good Lord had created, but even more fun was watching David's intensity as he saw the whole thing take place. I had never seen a dung beetle on our ranch before, but thanks to my son in diapers, and his mother, my life now had more marvel and more fun and more laughter.

72

David's Song of Joy and Acceptance Brings Laughter and Tears

O n this same trip, we were in the mobile home at the family ranch and, after we ate lunch, David waddled back and forth in his diapers, in the living room, singing as only a toddler can sing, "I adopted son. I adopted son" with great joy and smiles, and loving acceptance, on his face. Ever since he could understand English, we had told him that he was special, he was different from other children because we had picked him out for adoption, he wasn't just born to us, we had selected him, and that made him special.

As soon as he began to understand this, he made up his own song about it. We both laughed and cried as we heard him sing.

Laughter and tears often go together.

Later, when David had a more adult understanding of what adoption was, he once said, "There was a woman who didn't want me."

"Oh no," we replied. "Once there was a young woman who knew she was not able to raise you, so she carried you to full term, gave birth to you, and because she loved you and wanted you to have both a mother and a father who were able to take care of you, she had the doctor find us."

It was difficult for me to see David struggle through the facts about his adoption, but it also made me love him more and try to nurture him even more. Tears are indeed often linked to laughter.

73

Elizabeth Irene Cobb: the Raccoon, the Fawn, and the Copperhead Snake

Ever since we purchased *La Tierra de la Paz* ranch in northwest Bourbon County, on the Little Osage River that flows into Lake of the Ozarks, I had prayed that our children would love and enjoy the beauty of those rolling hills, the oak filled valleys, and the tall grass prairies.

Once, when Elizabeth was in early grade school, she went with me on a hike up the creek. We sat down on a fallen tree to rest. Because we were sitting quietly, a raccoon, who was taking a protein "range cube" I had left for the cattle, brought it down the hill and began eating it near us.

It was one of those magical moments I will treasure until the day I die remembering the look of awe on Elizabeth's face. The next morning, when she was still asleep, I quietly woke her so she could get up and see a doe and her newborn fawn come down the hill right near us.

Later, she wanted to help me move small concrete blocks from a shed that had fallen down. I was in front of her, carrying a couple of blocks and she was behind me, carrying one, when I heard her say, "Daddy."

I turned and told her to stand still. "Don't move."

She immediately stopped. After she had picked up her block, and was starting to follow me, a two foot long copperhead snake had come out of a hole from under the block. It slowly slid up over her shoe. It then slid past me and went down a second hole.

"Wow, Elizabeth," I said. "I am so glad your mother did not see that," and we both laughed.

Copperhead snake bites won't kill you, but they will make you pretty sick.

Elizabeth and I still have fun and laugh every time we talk about the raccoon, the fawn, and the copperhead snake. We all can have fun and laughter long after similar events. Systematically do this to have better mental health. Elizabeth still continues to enjoy God's creation with her friend Zack. Now she tells me her own stories of being with him outdoors.

Such stories help us to regularly reframe our lives in healthy ways whenever we make the decision to remember them.

74

Mindfulness and Fun and Laughter

Many people in recovery have a racing mind. A large part of recovery is learning how to slow down. Thomas Keating, Native American Holy Men and women, and many others, have taught me how to slow down and to live in the present moment, to savor each bite of food, note the taste, realize that every bite has a slightly different taste, enjoy each breath of air, take air in mindfully, release air mindfully, appreciate each heartbeat, live in the present moment, and relish the beauty in everything you see. It is something I have to cognitive remember every single day.

When we rush through life we exist, but we don't fully live. Totally listen to the words of your friend, rather than be thinking of how to reply. Savor every good moment and every difficult moment. Accept life on life's terms. Have fun watching the calves frolic through a pasture. Laugh with the kitten zipping through the living room as it exuberates in the sheer delight of simply being alive.

75

Fun and Laughter
as the Unseen World Opens

I was taking an afternoon nap when I heard my wife call my name. Waking up from a deep sleep, I found she was not anywhere in the house. At that moment, she started texting me from 40 miles away. How cool.

I prayed for a friend especially hard one day and, later, told them about it, only to learn that, at the precise time, they really needed prayer. Thousands of miles away I texted a friend I had not heard from in weeks. He wrote back, "Are you psychic? How did you know I have been going through a difficult time?"

How fun is that? What joy to sense the presence of God in the corner of a meadow or a clearing in the forest. What fun to write down a vivid dream and later discover it was a directive from God and from our own subconscious. A question I always ask those close to me, "Where does the Spirit of God begin and your own subconscious end?" It is a mystery.

What joy in watching someone recover from a terminal illness to the point that they outlive their physician who diagnosed them. What deep laughter in buying a ranch because I sensed the presence of God there and, many years later, be led "by chance" to a white-haired old gentlemen who grew up there.

"Did you ever hear about Elder Dizmang?" the old man said. "He was my grandfather. He started several churches in this region. He often came to see me when I was growing up here."

No wonder the ranch felt holy, it had been blessed by a man of God visiting his grandson many years ago.

A very deep source of fun and laughter in recovery can be found in opening up to the spirituality of the unseen world, a world which will be there forever.

76

Fun and Laugher like a Child:
Running, and Laughing, and Playing

I was at my health club, lying on a mat, doing Tai Chi, physical therapy stretches and Yoga, and limbering up before I worked out. It was a snowy winter day outside and I was in the soccer/baseball area of my gym. Two early grade school children, a boy and a girl, were playing with their older brother, throwing and kicking a soccer ball. It was a very big room so I just focused on getting more flexible. Their running and screaming and laughter had a sense of total abandonment and sheer pleasure. I was glad they were having fun. I was halfway into my regimen, and flat on my back, when the soccer ball hit me square on the left side of my face.

Without an apology, the three children put the ball away and left the gym quickly. I did not react, did not even look up at them, but continued to get ready for heavier exercise. The slap of the soccer ball on my head did get my attention. It made me think.

I began to see the sheer joy they exhibited for the ten to fifteen minutes they were playing and running and laughing. I realized that to have fun and laughter in recovery, we each must become like a little child. We must put away our adult pseudo-sophistication, because, after all, we each remain little boys and little girls deep inside during our entire lifetimes. Why not run and laugh and play as long as we can? Why not live with a sense of total abandonment? Why not take great delight in simple pleasures?

77

A Wrong Turn in the
Darkness of an Ozark Mountain Cave

My non-commissioned officer and I were working with young soldiers in a basic training battalion at Fort Leonard Wood, Missouri, affectionately and accurately called "Fort Lost in the Woods." When we finally got a day off, he suggested we explore a large cave in the forest beyond the east entrance of the Fort.

We got old battle dress uniforms on, because we knew we were going to get pretty dirty in the cave, and climbed up the mountain to the cave entrance, carrying our flashlights.

The cave opening was an awesome thirty feet high and thirty feet wide. There was a beautiful creek coming out of the cave. When we entered, several pigeons that nested there flew off. It was a hot and humid summer day, and we could feel the refreshing coolness from deep within the mountain flowing out of the cave entrance, down onto the valley floor.

At first we could walk upright on the damp clay floor but, as the cave got lower and lower, we had to hunch down to avoid hitting our heads. Not long afterwards, bending down in total darkness, I noticed, from the light of our flashlights, that, to our right, a side branch of the cave led somewhat downhill.

We continued on up a gradual incline. The cave got narrower and narrower until finally, we had to crawl on our hands and knees. Then it reached the point where, to get through, into a larger chamber, we had to get flat on our stomach on the damp clay floor, and slither through, like snakes.

When we stood up in the chamber, we could see that the celling had collapsed years ago and there was a pile of rubble about 20 feet high we would have to climb over in order to continue.

I asked my sergeant if he wanted to go further, and he said he did not. He led the way back toward the cave entrance. When we came to where the cave branched out to the left and to the right, he started to go down the left side. I told him that we did not come in that way, but he was adamant that it was the right way.

"Okay," I said. "I will sit here and wait for you at this juncture, because I am pretty sure you will come back."

I got an uneasy feeling in my stomach, sitting in total darkness, watching his light fade off. *Was I right or was he right?* I wondered. *Will he come back?* I shut off my light and waited.

Quite a few minutes passed before I saw his light turn a corner and start coming back toward me.

"Do you remember that creek coming out of the cave entrance?" he asked. "I was underneath that creek and I could not get out. I am going to follow you out."

When we finally got back to the light of the cave entrance, we stood there laughing. He had been lost. We had been in total darkness, but now we were in the light and heat of summer again, and we were covered with the damp clay of the cave floor. We were quite a sight.

Often in life we go down the wrong path and get lost, but if we turn back to the light and then stand in that light, and remember the darkness, we can laugh at our own stupidity and we can laugh at the darkness in our past.

Laughing at our past mistakes and making healthy fun of them, is such good mental hygiene.

78

Staying in the Light

Bruce Ames and I had canoed for years throughout the Ozark Mountains and Minnesota and Canada. When he retired, he kept calling me and asking me to go with him to northern Peru. He spoke Spanish and had been there before. He knew I spoke a little Spanish as well. After three years, I realized that maybe God was speaking to me to go with him, so we began a very interesting two week adventure.

We had to take two long overnight bus trips on narrow roads, often hanging over huge cliffs to get up to 10,000 feet. On the way I prayed. I knew several Native American Holy Men in the United States, so I prayed to be led to a Native American Holy Man in the mountains of northern Peru. Bruce and I, and John Zibell, were going to visit several Native American holy places there.

Our guide was Ernesto Cano Vilca. He was a 16th generation Holy Man. Not knowing who I was or what I did, he spilled out his compelling story to me as we drove to the first holy place.

Ernesto had been on a spiritual quest even as a child. His entrepreneurial parents were both very busy and so he decided to read everything he could find.

"Books were my companions and friends," he said. "I would watch other children running around outside, playing games, but that was not for me. I was not good in sports so I read and read."

Ernesto was 16th in a line of South American Indian family line of over fifteen generations of healers and native Holy Men and women. His parents took him to church and his grandmother taught him native teachings.

"When I was ill my *abuela* (grandmother) would give me special foods and plants, and I would get better. I still remember all the things she taught me."

As a teenager, he gradually eased away from spirituality, but he continued reading. I was amazed at his encyclopedic knowledge of the world. He began playing with a heavy metal band whose repertoire was the dark, satanic music of the American band called *Black Sabbath*. His band was popular in Peru. The band then went on a twenty day tour in neighboring Bolivia.

"I was drinking so much that I only remember three of those twenty days. This was my darkest time. I felt nothing but blackness. I had a vision where I was deep inside a dark mountain. I had a crown on my head, but I could not get out. Then I had my first good vision. I saw a small point of light in the darkness. The light opened up and I was standing before Jesus stretched out on the cross. He told me I was in darkness because I had not followed him. Then he pulled one hand off the cross and then the other off the cross. He reached out and held me tightly in his arms. It was then I quit drinking and turned toward the light. Now I try to help other people."

There are some very real teaching points in Ernesto's story: Fight the darkness. Stay in the light. Every day walk in light. Know where you are going. While you have the light, stay in the light and be that light to others. In the light of being healthy and clean and sober, and in recovery, fun and laughter will come.

Turning from Darkness to the Light, Ernesto Cano Vilca of Chachapoyas, Peru, reminds me of the scripture: *"Walk while you have the light so that darkness may not overtake you. If you walk in the dark you do not know where you are going."*

While you have the light, believe in the light. John 12:35-36

I have come as light into the world that whoever believes in me shall not abide in darkness. John 12:46, Jesus of Nazareth, the *Message Bible.*

POSTLUDE

It is my sincere hope that you will find a full recovery from any trauma, mental health issues, substance abuse, or physical health issues in your life by using these true stories to begin the process of reframing your life in the direction of having more fun and laughter.

Fun and laughter need not be shallow, temporary emotions, but rather a long-term decision by you to enjoy life, to relish every breath, and, to the utmost, live fully alive.

You are a child of God.

You belong in the world.

You are loved.

Have fun.

Exult in life.

Laugh a lot.

Have a thankful heart.

You deserve it.

OTHER ARTICLES, BOOKS, AND RESEARCH by Ronald Lee Cobb

George Fox and His Contributions to Seventeen Century Quaker Life and thought

The Quaker-Baptist Controversy in Seventeen Century England

The Theology of the Inner Self in the Writings of Alexander Solzhenitsyn

Russian Culture and Religion as Seen in the Writings of Alexander Solzhenitsyn

Guthrie Mound and the Hanging of John Guthrie

A Critical Evaluation of an Ecumenical Ministry to Senior Adults

Native American Spirituality as a Tool for Recovery from Alcohol and Drug Addiction

What to do when a Colleague has an Alcohol or Drug Problem

Memories of Bosnia: The 35th Divisions SFOR 13 NATO Peacekeeping Mission

Islam, What You Need to Know in the Twenty-First Century, a Primer for Peace

Spiritual Journeys: Life, Miracles, Power, and Love

www.ingramcontent.com/pod-product-compliance
Lightning Source LLC
Chambersburg PA
CBHW060046210326
41520CB00009B/1287